Bariatric Surgery - Past and Present

Edited by Burhan Hakan Kanat, Nizamettin Kutluer and Serhat Doğan

Published in London, United Kingdom

Bariatric Surgery - Past and Present
http://dx.doi.org/10.5772/intechopen.100966
Edited by Burhan Hakan Kanat, Nizamettin Kutluer and Serhat Doğan

Contributors
Ivaylo Tzvetkov, Asad Ullah, Juaquito M. Jorge, Frederick M. Tiesenga, Athanasios G. Pantelis, Awadh Alqahtani, Mohammad Almayouf, Rosa del Campo, Natalia Bastón-Paz, Manuel Ponce-Alonso, José Avendaño, María Garriga, Izzet Ulker, Elham Foroudi Pourdeh, Burhan Hakan Kanat, Muhammed Said Dalkılıç, Mehmet Gençtürk, Merih Yılmaz, Hasan Erdem, Selim Sözen, Abdullah Şişik

First published in London, United Kingdom, 2023 by IntechOpen
IntechOpen is the global imprint of INTECHOPEN LIMITED, registered in England and Wales, registration number: 11086078, 5 Princes Gate Court, London, SW7 2QJ, United Kingdom

British Library Cataloguing-in-Publication Data
A catalogue record for this book is available from the British Library

Additional hard and PDF copies can be obtained from orders@intechopen.com

Bariatric Surgery - Past and Present
Edited by Burhan Hakan Kanat, Nizamettin Kutluer and Serhat Doğan
p. cm.
Print ISBN 978-1-80356-320-6
Online ISBN 978-1-80356-321-3
eBook (PDF) ISBN 978-1-80356-322-0

Meet the editors

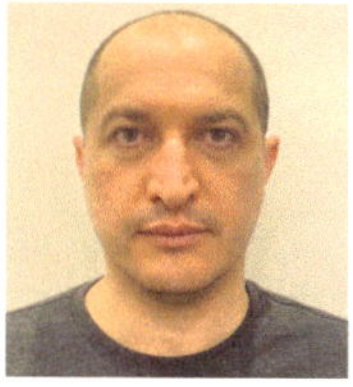

Dr. Burhan Hakan Kanat graduated from the Faculty of Medicine, İnönü University, Turkey, in 2005. He trained in general surgery at the Faculty of Medicine, Fırat University, Turkey, in 2011. He also worked as a specialist at the Elazığ Training and Research Hospital in Turkey. In 2013, he received a Certificate of Surgical Competence from the Turkish Surgery Society. He completed liver transplantation surgery at İnönü University in 2014–2015 and received training in breast-endocrine surgery in 2016. Dr. Kanat also worked at the Department of General Surgery, Faculty of Medicine, Health Sciences University, Turkey, as an associate professor from 2017 to 2020. Since October 2020, he has worked as an associate professor in the Department of General Surgery, Faculty of Medicine, Malatya Turgut Özal University, Turkey. He is a member of the Turkish Surgical Society, International Pilonidal Society, and Turkish Society of Colon and Rectal Surgery. Dr. Kanat is the author of more than 100 publications including 10 book chapters. He is also a review board member for several journals.

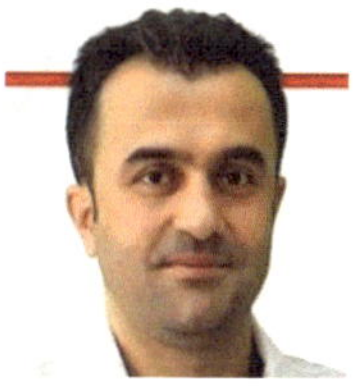

Dr. Nizamettin Kutluer graduated from the Faculty of Medicine, Fırat University, Turkey, in 2004. In 2011, he received general surgery training at Ankara Dışkapı Yıldırım Beyazıt Training and Research Hospital in Turkey. He first worked as a surgical specialist at Yerköy State Hospital, Turkey, in 2012. Then, in 2014, he worked as a general surgery specialist at Elazığ Training and Research Hospital, Turkey. He studied obesity and metabolic surgery at Elazig Fırat University, Turkey. Dr. Kutluer has been working as a general surgery specialist at Elazığ Private Eastern Anatolia Hospital, Turkey, since 2020.

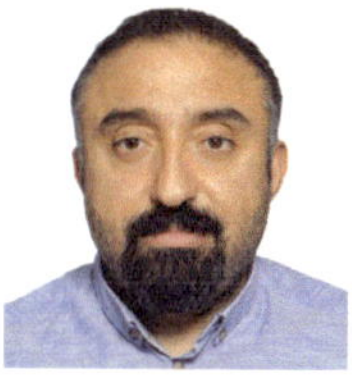

Dr. Serhat Doğan graduated from the Faculty of Medicine, Erciyes University, Turkey, in 2008. He trained in general surgery at the Faculty of Medicine, Necmettin Erbakan University, Meram Medicine School Konya, Turkey, in 2015. He also worked as a specialist at the Malatya Training and Research Hospital in Turkey. Since October 2021, he has worked as an assistant professor at the Department of General Surgery, Faculty of Medicine, Malatya Turgut Özal University, Turkey. Dr. Doğan is a member of the Turkish Surgical Society and an author of more than twenty publications including six book chapters. He is also a review board member for several journals.

Contents

Preface

Obesity is a complex and chronic disease with an increasing prevalence [1]. Bariatric surgery produces successful results in cases where physical activity, diet, and other medical treatments have failed. All types of bariatric surgery have their own advantages and disadvantages.

The word bariatrics is formed by the combination of the Greek word "-bar," which expresses weight, and "-iatria," which expresses treatment [2]. According to historical records, the first bariatric surgery was performed in Spain in the 10th century. The king of Leon, Sacho, was operated on by Ibn Shaprut, the doctor of the time, to lose weight. His method was quite simple and interesting. Sharput pricked the king's lips and left only enough space to drink soup and other liquids with a straw, helping the king to lose weight. This is the first bariatric surgery recorded in history [3].

Metabolic surgery was first introduced by Dr. Arnold Kremen in 1954 who performed jejunoileal bypass on dogs [4]. In 1966, University of Iowa's Dr. Edward E. Mason noted that patients who underwent subtotal gastrectomy for cancer lost significant weight. Dr. Mason suggested the first "bariatric surgery" and performed the first gastric bypass [5].

In 1976, Dr. Nicola Scopinaro developed biliopancreatic diversion [BPD], a maladaptive procedure to treat obesity [6]. Later, Dr. Picard Marceau reported duodenal switch as an alternative to BPD [7].

In the 1980s, Dr. Mason began to use vertical banded gastroplasty [VBG] [8]. In 1986, Dr. Lubomyr Kuzmak developed a horizontal gastric band [9]. In 1992, Dr. Guy-Bernard Cadière placed a laparoscopic gastric band [10]. The number of surgeries performed with the laparoscopic technique has increased steadily since its inception.

Sleeve gastrectomy is another bariatric surgery technique that has become widespread in recent years. It was developed in the late 1990s by Dr. Michel Gagner who showed that sufficient weight can be lost with sleeve gastrectomy [11].

This book presents a history of bariatric surgery, examines current bariatric techniques, and discusses the exciting future of this procedure, including surgical robots, robotic coding, gene therapy, and more.

I wish to thank to my co-editors Dr. Nizamettin Kutluer and Dr. Serhat Doğan.

Burhan Hakan Kanat and Serhat Doğan
Malatya Turgut Ozal University Medicine School,
Department of General Surgery,
Malatya, Turkey

Nizamettin Kutluer
Special East Anatolian Hospital,
Department of General Surgery,
Elazig, Turkey

References

[1] https://www.who.int/health-topics/obesity#tab=tab_1 / [Erişim Tarihi: 4.12.2022]

[2] Berdanier CD, Dwyer JT, Feldman EB. Handbook of Nutrition and Food. Boca Raton, London, New York: CRC Press; 2007. p. 1247

[3] Gargantilla Madera P, Arroyo Pardo N. Hasday: tratamiento dela obesidad en el siglo x. Endocrinología y Nutrición. 2016;**63**:100-101

[4] Kremen AJ, Linner JH, Nelson CH. An experimental evaluation of the nutritional importance of proximal and distal small intestine. Annals of Surgery. 1954;**140**:439-448

[5] Mason EE, Ito C. Gastric bypass in obesity. Surgical Clinics of North America. 1967;**47**:1345-1351

[6] Scopinaro N, Gianetta E, Civalleri D, Bonalumi U, Bachi V. Bilio-pancreatic bypass for obesity: II. Initial experience in man. British Journal of Surgery. 1979;**66**:618-620

[7] Marceau P, Biron S, Bourque R, Potvin M, Hould F, Simard S. Biliopancreatic diversion with a new type of gastrectomy. Obesity Surgery. 1993;**3**:29-35. DOI: 10.1381/096089293765559728

[8] Mason EE. Vertical banded gastroplasty for obesity. Archives of Surgery. [Chicago, Ill: 1960]. 1982;**117**:701-706

[9] Kuzmak L. A review of seven years' experience with silicone gastric banding. Obesity Surgery. 1991;**1**:403-408. DOI: 10.1381/096089291765560809

[10] Cadiere GB, Bruyns J, Himpens J, Favretti F. Laparoscopic gastroplasty for morbid obesity. British Journal of Surgery. 1994;**81**:1524

[11] Ren CJ, Patterson E, Gagner M. Early results of laparoscopic biliopancreatic diversion with duodenal switch: a case series of 40 consecutive patients. Obesity Surgery. 2000;**10**:514-523. DOI: 10.1381/096089200321593715

Section 1

Bariatric Surgery

Chapter 1

Do All Bariatric Surgery Methods Have the Same Effects on the Gut Microbiota?

Elham Foroudi Pourdeh and Izzet Ulker

Abstract

Despite the various treatment methods that exist for obesity, the most effective treatment for long-term weight control is bariatric surgery. Different surgical methods affect different mechanisms, such as appetite change, restriction of intake, and control of hunger. Divert food from the proximal part of the small intestine, food aversion, increased energy expenditure, malabsorption of macronutrients, and modifications of bile aside profiles and the gut microbiota. Gut microbiota plays an important role in maintaining human health. Dysbiosis usually has detrimental effects and may also have long-term consequences that lead to diseases or disorders, such as diabetes, obesity, and inflammatory bowel disease. While Firmicutes are abundant in the gut microbiota of obese individuals, Bacteroidetes are more abundant in individuals with normal weight. Thus, specific changes in the gut microbial composition are associated with obesity. The suggestion of growing evidence of bariatric surgery's success is because of the procedure's effect on the gut microbiota. Bariatric surgery changes the short-chain fatty acids composition by certain changes in the gut microbiota, thus affecting host metabolism, including intestinal hormone secretion and insulin sensitivity. Different methods of bariatric surgery alter the gut microbiota differently.

Keywords: bariatric surgery, gut microbiota

1. Introduction

Bariatric surgery is the name given to surgical methods to control obesity [1]. There are varying treatment methods for obesity, such as lifestyle modification (which includes behavioral modification, increased physical activity, and caloric restriction), pharmacotherapy, and bariatric surgery [2]. The main obesity treatment method is weight loss through lifestyle interventions. These interventions include diet and exercise. However, in most cases, with these measures, sufficient weight loss is not achieved, and gaining weight is common and does not lead to a significant and lasting solution. The use of medications is another possible approach, although their effectiveness may seem limited [3]. There are few effective treatment options for severe obesity. For severe obesity, the most effective treatment for long-term weight control in adults is bariatric surgery [3, 4]. Bariatric surgery methods in general are considered safe. The average preoperative mortality is less than 3% [5]. Bariatric surgery is recommended for adults with excessive obesity (BMI ≥ 40 kg/m2) or those obese with BMI ≥ 35 kg/m2 in attendance of at least one significant comorbidity caused by obesity. The health risks that interact with obesity are hypertension, type 2 diabetes mellitus, stroke, coronary heart disease, asthma, obstructive sleep apnea, and osteoarthritis, among other health complications [2]. The different surgeries methods effects assorted mechanisms, including change of appetite, restriction of intake, control of hunger, divert food from the proximal part of the small intestine, food aversion, increased energy expenditure, malabsorption of macronutrients, and modifications of bile aside profiles and the gut microbiota. Choosing the surgical methods depends on the surgeon or patient preference, permanent anatomical change, and accessibility for proper aftercare. Nowadays, bariatric surgery contains three main types of methods. They are categorized according to their mechanism: A) Restrictive methods, aimed at reducing the size of the stomach to restrict solids consumption include gastric imbrication, sleeve gastrectomy (SG), and adjustable gastric banding (LAGB) B) Malabsorptive methods, by shortening the small intestine, thus surface area exposed to food is reduced and the absorption of nutrients is reduced, include jejunoileal bypass (JIB) C) Combined malabsorptive and respective methods include the Biliopancreatic diversion (BPD) [3]. The most common bariatric surgery methods are laparoscopic, which include sleeve gastrectomy (SG) and Roux-en-Y gastric bypass (RYGB). In terms of popularity, sleeve gastrectomy has surpassed Roux-en-Y gastric bypass in the last few years [2].

2. Bariatric surgery methods

2.1 Roux-en-Y gastric bypass (RYGB)

The surgical treatment that is still considered a standard technique and widely used for the treatment of morbid obesity is RYGB [6, 7]. In RYGB, a small gastric pouch attaches to the small intestine and bypasses the stomach, duodenum, and proximal jejunum [8]. Recently, RYGB is the second most common operation worldwide, sleeve gastrectomy (SG) preceded that [9]. Although RYGB frequency is surpassed worldwide by sleeve gastrectomy (SG), long-term results in weight reduction, remission of comorbidities also changing quality of life, are well documented and make the RYGB a common bariatric procedure [6, 7, 10]. For these good results, identifiable factors are mostly a combination of mechanisms of action, which include mild malabsorption by bypassing a reasonable part of the jejunum, mechanical restriction of calorie intake due to the small gastric pouch, and hormonal changes like a decrease in the production of ghrelin, early secretion of PYY and changes in various incretin levels, such as GLP1 [11]. For patients with gastroesophageal reflux disease, many are seen as the gold standard treatment and it is recommended as the first method of choice for patients with type 2 diabetes mellitus [12]. Hepatic hypersensitivity to insulin has been shown to improve within a week after RYGB, and after months, after major weight loss, insulin sensitivity in adipose tissue and skeletal muscle also improves [13]. However, due to changes in intestinal anatomy after LRYGB, the internal hernia can occur through the Petersen space mesenteric defect or the mesenteric jejunojonostomy defect during follow-up [10]. After LRYGB, a frequent complication is small bowel obstruction [14]. Fasting bile acid levels increase after RYGB but do not increase after SG [15]. Long-term complications may occur. Re-interventions are sometimes needed. In very rare cases, a return to normal anatomy may be due to severe dumping syndrome, gastric bypass malnutrition, excessive weight loss, postprandial hypoglycemia, or recurrent marginal ulcers [9]. Long-term complications, such as anemia, may not be diagnosed by non-bariatric specialists. Anemia causes include folate, iron, and B12 deficiency. Bleeding marginal ulcers, and selenium, copper, and vitamin A deficiency are the less common causes [16].

2.2 Laparoscopic sleeve gastrectomy (LSG)

The most common bariatric surgery, which is performed is sleeve gastrectomy (SG) [17]. Some advantages include intact and normal intestinal absorption, preservation of pylorus preventing dumping syndrome, technical efficiency, and the first appropriate step for extremely obese patients [18]. Additional benefits, such as maintaining gastrointestinal integrity and preventing malabsorption [19]. The extreme objective of the method is to evacuate between 60 and 70% of the stomach, counting the fundus, leaving a long, thin banana-shaped stomach [17, 18]. Narrowing of the gastric leads to significant limitations of stomach capacity also in other metabolic modifications. Ghrelin is one of the hormones that increments and stimulates the patient's appetite. It is produced by cells found within the fundus. Resection of the fundus significantly diminished the basal level of ghrelin, diminishing appetite in patients who experienced LSG [18]. PYY increased postoperatively and leptin, insulin and ghrelin decreased. Probably due to improved beta-cell function and improved insulin sensitivity, insulin levels decreased following LSG. Also, decreased postoperative leptin levels may be related to decreased leptin resistance or improved leptin sensitivity [20]. LSG has illustrated its effectiveness in accomplishing weight loss and determination of obesity-related comorbidities; the concept of SG is simple, but performing incorrectly some components can cause serious complications [18]. Bleeding, staple line leak, stenosis, venous thromboembolism, intra-abdominal abscess, gastroesophageal reflux, and strictures are complications associated with LSG [17]. Staple line leakage and bleeding are the major complications in the early postoperative period. The most common complication, which occurs in about 1.1–8.7% of cases, is staple line bleeding. The most life-threatening and dangerous complication is leakage of staple line with 0.5%-2.7 incidence ranging [21]. The potential causes of leakage are a technical failure, a stapler's mechanical failure, functionality and the shape of the sleeve, high intraluminal pressure, incisura angularis obstruction, or poor wound healing [19]. Primary subphrenic abscess and secondary rupture of the diaphragm, which can rarely be caused by gastric leakage, eventually will lead to gastrobronchial fistula. Gastrobronchial fistula is a chronic gastric leakage late complication located above the staple line [22]. Compared to laparoscopic adjustable gastric banding (LAGB), a very popular method over a decade before, sleeve gastrectomy is a simple yet powerful metabolic operation that changes the eating behavior, gut functions, and glycemic control by activating hormonal pathways, and the procedure needs no foreign implant. And compared to RYGB, it is technically easier and does not require intestinal anastomosis. The LSG is limited to the stomach and prevents the presence of an internal hernia in postoperative follow-up [23].

2.3 Laparoscopic adjustable gastric banding (LAGB)

One of the most secure surgical methods used to treat obesity is LAGB [24]. Firstly, in 1993, laparoscopic adjustable gastric banding was described by Belachew. Since then, the LAGB has undergone many changes, revisions, and corrections to become the way it is now defined. These changes influenced both surgical and technological techniques, but most importantly, the management of pre-and postoperative [25].

In LAGB, a silicone ring is placed around the gastric to create a little upper stomach pouch under the esophagus. Within the 1970s, this method was introduced and remains secure, well endured, and effective with a relatively low risk of complications. Increasing the effect of weight loss without compromising safety by adjusting the band is another benefit of this method. An option that makes LAGB attractive to most patients is that it is a reversible form of laparoscopic surgery, although it is not touted as a temporary method due to the considerable risk of regaining weight after removal [24]. LAGB at first accounted for most methods and affected weight loss by a restrictive mechanism [26]. And indeed even though its popularity has been diminishing over time, it remains a choice for a specific group of patients, creating significant weight loss and improving obesity-associated comorbidities [24]. Due to the lack of any resection or anastomosis, reversibility, low life-threatening complications, and a minimally invasive intervention, LAGB surgical procedure seems to be useful [27]. Obesity to a lower degree, at a younger age, and at the time of surgery, the lesser severity of comorbidities for successful weight loss can be an important indicator, making these patients the perfect candidate for LAGB [24]. LAGB is the simplest form of minimally invasive or surgical method performed for obesity, but it is less commonly used due to the high rate of secondary revision to complications and late weight gain. Weight loss was promising in the initial results but in the long-term, the result is less encouraging [28]. LAGB has some minor complications, such as port slippage, port tube separation, and port infection, and major complications, such as band intolerance, band erosion, band migration, pouch enlargement, band slippage, and band opening [27]. One of the less common late-onset complications is digestive lumen band erosion/migration, which occurs after LAGB. Late complications after LAGB are more than the initial complications and include band slippage, device-related complications, band erosion, and pouch dilation. Major life-threatening complications, manifesting as severe gastrointestinal hemorrhage, perforation, or obstruction are rare and require immediate surgical intervention [28].

2.4 Biliopancreatic diversion (BPD)

One of the most effective surgical methods for obesity is BPD, which generally loses more than 72% of excess body weight in 5 years. Firstly, Scopinaro described BPD, done over the past 25 years, and lead to sustainable and effective long-term weight loss [29]. Among the existing bariatric methods, biliopancreatic diversion (BPD) was common in prior decades. It is a combination of a Roux-en-Y construction with a distal gastrectomy [30]. Biliary and pancreatic juices are transported by the biliopancreatic limb to the common limb, while ingested food is transferred to the common limb by the alimentary limb [30]. One of the most effective methods in decreasing comorbidities of obesity and weight loss with minimal long-term weight regain is biliopancreatic diversion (BPD) [30, 31]. Patients lose weight because of the reduction in the area of absorption by bypassing most of the intestines with nutrients, also because of reduced absorption and digestion by the attachment of nutrients to the biliopancreatic enzymes and secretions distally [32]. BPD leads to many metabolic syndrome complications remission [29]. BPD has a positive effect on T2DM and other complications of metabolic syndrome in the short-term and long-term. After surgery, triglycerides, total cholesterol, and LDL decrease, while HDL levels increase. HTN improvement or resolution is observed. Before surgery, the HTN incidence was 56.7%. After surgery, approximately 50% of hypertensive patients improved or recovered after a one-year follow-up [31]. Signaling of bile acid, increased secretion of intestinal hormones (oxyntomodulin, PYY, and GLP-1), Gut microbiota changing and intestinal glucose transport reduction through circulating branched-chain amino acids and SGLT1, improved initial sensitivity and secretion of insulin, and increased satiety, is thought to cause these effects [29]. However, BPD is not widespread due to it is associated with long-term side effects, such as vitamin deficiency and protein malnutrition due to malabsorption [29, 31]. BPD anatomical late complications were reported to a less frequent [29]. Protein malnutrition is a common and frightening aspect of bariatric surgery [31]. In 7.7–11.9% of patients with BPD, protein malnutrition can occur; when the gastric pouch is less than 200 MLS, this reaches even in 17.8%. To minimize this risk, the common limb's length and the gastric pouch's size can be adapted (increase from 50 cm to 100 cm). In 60% of BPD patients, iron deficiency anemia will occur due to exclusion of the proximal jejunum and duodenum and decreased gastric acid secretion [29]. Especially, according to the fat-soluble vitamins in malabsorptive bariatric methods, multiple vitamin supplements will be required. Calcium metabolism changes significantly, usually due to vitamin D deficiency. Weight loss, even before surgery, reduces bone density because of mechanical disorders of load on bones and usually, secondary hyperparathyroidism is established. Vitamin D and calcium deficiency occur more often after malabsorptive methods than in restrictive methods [31]. BPD, which is surgically challenging, is rarely performed today due to the high risk of lifelong needs and nutritional complications for follow-up [29]. Presently, late complications are frequently observed in elderly patients [30].

3. Gut microbiota

There are trillions of microorganisms in the human body and the coordinated function of these microorganisms is important for the host life. The population of microorganisms in the intestine reaches its highest density. This complex microbial community that forms in the intestinal is the gut microbiota [33]. There are 100 trillion microorganisms in the human intestine. The gut microbiota is mainly formed by five phyla and populations, while the intestine is dominated by bacterial species (phyla Firmicutes and Bacteriodetes). There are also viruses, bacteria, archaea, fungi, phages, nematodes, and protists. There is a symbiotic relationship between microorganisms and their human hosts. Through this symbiotic relationship, microorganisms protect and support the structure of the intestinal mucosa during their evolution. There are at least 150 times more genes in the gut microbiota than in the human genome. And it weighs approximately 1 to 2 kg [34–36]. After birth, the ecosystem of gut microbiota is created by the transfer of maternal bacteria and environmental bacteria and continues to expand until adulthood [36]. Bacteria's quantity in the gastrointestinal tract increases from the proximal part to the distal parts. More than 70% of all body microorganisms are located in the large intestine, which is usually associated with host health and disease. In addition, the lumen has a higher bacterial diversity and the mucosal layer has a lower bacterial diversity [35]. Some environmental parameters that may affect the composition of the gastrointestinal microbiota are water activity, PH, availability of nutrients, oxygen levels, and temperature. The diverse and abundant members of the gut microbiota play an important role in maintaining human health by promoting host cell differentiation, by breaking down food to release nutrients that otherwise would be inaccessible to the host, modulating/stimulating the immune system, and preventing colonization by pathogens they protect the host [33]. The presence of large numbers of bacteria in the gastrointestinal tract causes metabolic activity and biochemical diversity that have interactions with the host physiology [35]. Many factors can shift the balance of gut microbiota, and thus, disrupt gut microbial homeostasis and cause dysbiosis. Dysbiosis usually has detrimental effects and may also have long-term consequences that lead to diseases or disorders, such as diabetes, obesity, and inflammatory bowel disease [33]. Dysbiosis is associated with three different phenomena that can occur simultaneously: losing beneficial organisms, potentially harmful bacteria overgrowth, and losing overall microbial diversity [34]. Bacteriocins, which inhibit the bacterial pathogens growing that cause dysbiosis by their antibacterial action are produced by Lactobacillus Plantarum and Lactobacillus para case [37]. For homeostasis and proper metabolic function gut microbiota's health is crucial. Changes in microbiota composition may lead to diabetes and obesity by affecting homeostasis and substantially altering host metabolism and affecting central appetite mechanisms [36]. Proteobacteria lead to metabolic diseases, such as obesity, because it is associated with dysbiosis [37]. Therefore, potentially new anti-obesity strategies may be proposed by modulating intestinal microbiota with fecal microbiota transplantation or dietary interventions, including probiotics and prebiotics. The suggestion of growing evidence of bariatric surgery's success is because of the procedure's effect on the gut microbiota. Bariatric surgery changes the short-chain fatty acids composition by particular changes in the gut microbiota. Thus, affecting host metabolism, including intestinal hormone secretion and sensitivity of insulin. While *Firmicutes* are abundant in the gut microbiota of obese individuals. *Bacteroidetes* are more abundant in individuals with normal BMI, which break down plant starches and plant fibers for energy, thus specific changes in the gut microbial composition are associated with obesity [36]. The increase in the genus *Lactobacillus*, which belongs to the *Firmicutes phylum* was associated with obesity [37]. For metabolic syndrome and obesity, the gut microbiota is an effective and potential factor. Gut microbiota can also affect insulin resistance and hyperglycemia, which are associated with obesity. The effect of intestinal microbiota on insulin and glucose homeostasis may be due to its effect on changing the relative abundance and composition of bile acid species [36]. Bacteria can produce major neurotransmitters. The microbiota also has the potential to affect other levels of neurotransmitters, including gasotransmitters, steroids, neuropeptides, endocannabinoids, and histamine among others [38]. Gut bacteria are involved in the production of neuroactive metabolites, including γ-aminobutyric acid (GABA) and serotonin, thereby affecting central appetite control. And by the effect on serotonin metabolism, which might also influence glucose homeostasis. The gut microbiota also may affect hepatic lipid metabolism, fat storage, and hepatic triglyceride storage. Some bacterial strains affect satiety and appetite by altering the secretion of gut hormones, including ghrelin, leptin, GLP-1, and PYY, through the hypothalamic neuroendocrine pathways. Gut microbiota by altering mood and modulating reward pathways might also affect feeding behavior. The main factor affecting the activity and composition of the microbiota is diet. The gut microbiota is directly shaped by the various components of the diet [36].

4. Effects of bariatric surgery methods on gut microbiota

4.1 Roux-en-Y gastric bypass (RYGB)-gut microbiota

Bariatric surgery modifies the gut microbiota. Bariatric surgery also affects the physiology of the distal intestine and has a great influence on activity and the composition of the gut microbiota. Different methods of bariatric surgery alter the intestinal microbiota differently [39]. Bacterial diversity and richness are restored by RYGB surgery, and the frequency of several groups of bacteria is significantly altered [40]. These changes after surgery may affect weight loss, weight maintenance, and metabolic improvement. They may also cause weight gain [40, 41]. Patients who lost weight successfully after RYGB surgery had a significant difference in gut microbiota compared to patients who showed weight regain [41]. Patient preferences for high-fat and high-carbohydrate foods decrease after RYGB surgery. Patients have reportedly lost motivation to eat. Another common effect of RYGB surgery is to alter the gut microbiota and its related metabolites. *Escherichia Coli, Streptococcus, pneumonia, Klebsiella, Akkermansia muciniphila*, *Dentium*, and *Bifidobacterium* in the feces of patients increased after RYGB surgery [42]. After RYGB surgery, there is a decrease in *Firmicutes* and an increase in the frequency of *Verrucomicrobia* (*Akkermansia*) and *proteobacteria* in patients. After surgery, the *phylum Bacteroidetes* abundance decreases. Also, there is a decrease in the genus *Clostridium* and abundance of *the Fusobacteriaceae* family. *Gammaproteobacteria* (including *Enterobacteriaceae*), and the genus *Succinivibrio* increased following RYGB. Also, after surgery in animals and humans, an increase in *Enterococcus* was observed. This genus competes for intestinal epithelium adherence, and hereby, prevents the colonization of pathogenic bacteria and also has anti-inflammatory effects by producing butyrate [41]. After RYGB, the pH of the intestinal is lower compared to SG. Excluded parts of digestive transit in RYGB are the distal stomach and small intestine. Therefore, avoided stomach acidity and in the intestine, hydrochloric acid is reduced. Some studies have shown the pH reduction effect in inhibiting *Bacteroidetes* growth in bacterial culture. pH is important in the distribution of fermentation end-products [39]. After RYGB, a decrease in gastric acid secretion causes the incompletely digested proteins to increment in the gut and this results in the production of putrescine. Bacteria of the genus *Klebsiella* that has increased after RYGB. Also, can produce putrescine. This polyamine is metabolized to GABA, which stimulates the GLP-1 levels increments and improves insulin resistance. Similarly, the genus *Lachnobacterium,* which increased after RYGB improves glucose homeostasis and insulin resistance via short-chain fatty acids [41]. Metabolites like short-chain fatty acids produced by the intestinal microbiota have a beneficial effect on health and they have been linked to glycemic improvement, food intake regulation, and weight loss [43]. When the obese diabetic patients' fecal microbiota is evaluated before and after RYGB surgery, and preoperatively increase in *desulfovibrio* levels is seen in patients who have no postoperative T2DM remission compared with patients who have metabolic improvement [44]. Species, such as *pneumonia, Klebsiella, Alistipes, muciniphila*, and *Akkermansia,* are species that are augmented after RYGB and their relative abundance is associated with reduced adiposity [45]. There is *Streptococcus* and *villanelle* increment and *Claudia decrement* (all belong to the *Firmicutes phylum*). These changes can have important clinical consequences after surgery. For example, *Streptococcus* and *Veillonella* metabolize lactate, which in turn affects butyrate metabolism and epithelial barrier integrity. Increasing the integrity of the intestinal epithelium can improve metabolic disorders and reduce low-grade systemic inflammation. *Akkermensia* contains mucin-destroying microbes and in several studies has been shown increment after bariatric surgery. According to previous animal studies, *Akkermensia muciniphila* has been shown to protect against diabetes and obesity by potentially reducing low-grade inflammation and endotoxemia, as well as enhancing the barrier of the intestinal epithelium. *Akkermensia muciniphila* in humans also was associated with improved insulin sensitivity markers.

A negative correlation has previously been reported between serum leptin and *E. Coli* after RYGB [43]. Reducing stomach volume, which is included in RYGB, dramatically reduces the amount of food intake. Individual changes in diet can alter gut microbiota and it should be considered when considering changes in gut microbiota after bariatric surgery procedures [44]. Hospital-associated pathogens, such as *pneumonia, Klebsiella*, and *clostridium*, perfringens have also been shown to increase after RYGB. After surgery, one of the reasons for opportunistic pathogens increments is the routine administration of operative prophylactic antibiotics and alternation of the gastrointestinal environment [43]. RYGB surgery procedure resulted in a significant reduction in estimated and observed fungal diversity and richness. This contradicts many reports of bacterial alpha diversity increments. Despite the unidirectional changes observed in bacterial microbiota, changes in fungal microbiota after RYGB are individual [40].

4.2 Laparoscopic sleeve gastrectomy (LSG)-gut microbiota

Changes in the composition of the gut microbial community after surgery can affect metabolic outcomes. In particular, SG alters certain gut bacteria's relative abundance. It leads to increases in the species that improve the phenotypes of diabetes and obesity, abundance. For obese mice, fecal transplantation from mice and human patients post-bariatric surgery has metabolic benefits, such as improved insulin sensitivity, glucose tolerance, and weight loss. Importantly, in mice, antibiotics abolish the SG effectiveness due to gut microbiota disruption. These findings increase the possibility that after SG in metabolic changes gut bacteria are involved. Gut bacteria communicate through the portal vein by transporting a bacterial-derived molecule from the intestine to the liver [46]. SG leads to persistent changes in the intestinal microbiome by decreasing dysbiosis due to an increase in *Bacteroidetes* and a decrease in *Firmicutes*. SG improves diurnal oscillation and dysbiosis and increases microbial richness [47]. Compared to before LSG the percentage of *Phylum Verrucomicrobia* significantly increased after 1 month and 6 months. Percentages for the *Streptococcaceae* family also significantly increased. Also, *Christensenellaceae* increased after 1 month and 3 months, *Verrucomicrobiaceae* increased after 1 month and 6 months, *Rikenellaceae* increased after 6 months, and *Fusobacteriaceae* increased after 2 weeks, *A. muciniphila* significantly increased after 1 month and 6 months. For gut microbiota, the diversity indices OS, PD, and Chao1 were significantly increased after 6 months. The percentage of *Mogibacteriaceae* family after 3 months and 6 months were significantly decreased than before LSG [48]. SG surgery does not affect the presence of *F. Prausnitzii*, a butyrate producer in feces. LRYGB resulted in a greater increase in oral colonizers (genus *Veillonela* and *Streptococcus*) than in SG. *A. Muciniphila*, which negatively correlated with inflammation, increases in a similar proportion in patients after LRYGB or SG. *E. Coli* increment may reflect gut and host adaptation to energy harvest maximization in the post-bariatric surgery starvation-like condition [49]. In a rodent model, it was shown that *A. Muciniphila* inhibited metabolic abnormalities and body fat accumulation. However, with decreasing biological parameters related to obesity, increasing diversity of α and other taxa like *the Rikenellaceae* family is more associated. Although not much attention has been paid to *Rikenellaceae*, the results suggest that *the Rikenellaceae* taxon may play a role in the metabolic benefits of LSG and weight loss [48]. Changes in the microbiome after SG, particularly the reduction of *Clostridia*, lead to a decrease in lithocholic acid (LCA) production, which ultimately leads to increased glucoregulatory compound CA7S production. Lithocolicacid (LCA) by inducing CA7S synthesis in murine liver and human hepatocytes affects host metabolism. After SG, the amount of lithocholic acid (LCA) that is transported from the intestine to the liver through the portal vein increases. LCA induces colonic acid sulfonation and activates vitamin D receptors both *in vivo* in mice and *in vitro* in human hepatocytes. CA7S synthesized by LCA in human hepatocytes can induce the secretion of GLP-1 in enteroendocrine cells and provides a link between the changes in BA observed after SG and the surgery's metabolic benefits [46]. After LSG, *Fusobacteriaceae* and *Streptococcaceae* families relative abundance increased. These species are thought to have a pathogenic property, such as colorectal carcinogenic risk. They may be high due to reduced gastric passage time and decreased gastric juice secretion by LSG. After LSG, although the α diversity index is restored, the total number of gut microbiota remains lower than in healthy individuals. Disorders, such as Parkinson's disease, colorectal cancer, and inflammatory bowel disease, are associated with decreased total microbiota [48]. *Pseudobutyrivibrio* and *Prevotella sp.* increase after SG, they can inhibit colon cancer cell formation [50]. *Clostridium* species became enriched after SG, while LRYGB harmed them, which suggests the intestine is still largely anaerobic after SG. In this regard, a higher ferredoxin oxidoreductase relative abundance was observed post-LRYGB compared to SG, which is associated generally with aerobic respiration [49]. After SG Microbiome changes may protect from progressive hypertension related to multiple strains of *Lactobacillus* [51]. After 9 years postoperatively, changes in gut microbiota are less pronounced in LSG patients versus RYGB patients [52].

4.3 Laparoscopic adjustable gastric banding (LAGB)-gut microbiota

To our knowledge gut microbiota changes, have not been studied after LAGB surgery [53].

4.4 Biliopancreatic diversion (BPD)-gut microbiota

BPD/DS rats have significantly different microbiota than SHAM animals. Decreased gut microbiota richness and diversity were observed in BPD/DS rats. Microbial profile analysis showed a major shift from presurgical Clostridiales-dominated microbiota to high-concentration microbiota in *Bifidobacteriales* soon after surgery. After BPD/SD, the gut is divided into three functional segments: the alimentary limb, biliopancreatic limb, and common limb. *Bifidobacteriales* have a high content in the alimentary limb and common limb. But because the biliopancreatic limb contains a significant amount of *Actinomycetales*, it is different from the other two limbs. In BPD/DS, unlike RYGB, it was shown that *Bifidobacteriales* elevated significantly as represented by the increasing abundance of *the Bifidobacterium* genus. In the lower part of the intestine, the presence of nutrients, which is digestible, but undigested can change the microbiota. In BPD/SD rats, changes in the gut microbiota were associated with the beneficial influence of malabsorption procedures. Increasing the proportion of *Bifidobacteriales* bacteria associated with the genus *Bifidobacterium* may have health benefits for the host. *Bifidobacterium* predominance in the microbiota can reduce low-grade inflammation. The positive outcomes of surgery may be because of gut microbiota modulation and more specifically increase in *Bifidobacterium* abundance throughout the gastro-intestinal tract [54].

5. Conclusions

Although various surgical methods may have long-term side effects, they can lead to the improvement of obesity and its related disorders, and changes in the microbiota and related metabolites are effective in this matter. For example, bacteria of the genus Klebsiella, which has increased after RYGB, by producing putrescine and metabolizing This polyamine into GABA can increase the GLP-1 levels and improve insulin resistance. Similarly, the genus Lachnobacterium, which increased after RYGB improves glucose homeostasis and insulin resistance via short-chain fatty acids. Species, such as pneumonia, Klebsiella, Alistipes, muciniphila, and Akkermansia, are species that are augmented after RYGB and their relative abundance is associated with reduced adiposity. Also, SG leads to persistent changes in the intestinal microbiome by decreasing dysbiosis due to an increase in Bacteroidetes and a decrease in Firmicutes. Changes in gut microbiota are less pronounced in LSG patients versus RYGB patients. Also, The positive outcomes of BPD/SD surgery may be because of gut microbiota modulation and more specifically increase in Bifidobacterium abundance throughout the gastrointestinal tract. In BPD/DS, unlike RYGB, it was shown that Bifidobacteriales elevated significantly as represented by the increasing abundance of the Bifidobacterium genus.

Conflict of interest

The authors declare no conflict of interest.

Author details

Elham Foroudi Pourdeh[1] and Izzet Ulker[2]*

1 Departmant of Nutrition and Dietetics, Ataturk University, Health Sciences, Erzurum, Turkiye

2 Departmant of Nutrition and Dietetics, Erzurum Technical University, Health Sciences, Erzurum, Turkiye

*Address all correspondence to: izzetulker@gmail.com; izzet.ulker@erzurum.edu.tr

References

[1] Ámézquita GM, Baeza LC, Ríos EM, Francesetti MV, Rybertt VV, Gutiérrrez RM. Bariatric surgery in adolescents. Revista Chilena de Pediatría. 2019;**90**:17-25. DOI: 10.32641/rchped.v90i1.875

[2] Gasoyan H, Tajeu G, Halpern MT, Sarwer DB. Reasons for underutilization of bariatric surgery: The role of insurance benefit design. Surgery for Obesity and Related Diseases. 2019;**15**:146-151. DOI: 10.1016/j.soard.2018.10.005

[3] Cerreto M, Santopaolo F, Gasbarrini A, Pompili M, Ponziani FR. Bariatric surgery and liver disease: General considerations and role of the gut-liver Axis. Nutrients. 2021;**13**:2649. DOI: 10.3390/nu13082649

[4] Istfan NW, Lipartia M, Anderson WA, Hess DT, Apovian CM. Approach to the patient: Management of the Post-Bariatric Surgery Patient with Weight Regain. The Journal of Clinical Endocrinology and Metabolism. 2021;**106**:251-263. DOI: 10.1210/clinem/dgaa702

[5] Korakas E, Kountouri A, Raptis A, Kokkinos A, Lambadiari V. Bariatric surgery and type 1 diabetes: Unanswered questions. Front Endocrinology (Lausanne). 2020;**11**:525909. DOI: 10.3389/fendo.2020.525909

[6] Salminen P, Peterli R. Roux-en-Y gastric bypass limb lengths-how to optimize the balance between weight loss and risk of malnutrition? BJS Open. 2021;**5**. DOI: 10.1093/bjsopen/zrab120

[7] Chahal-Kummen M, Blom-Høgestøl IK, Eribe I, Klungsøyr O, Kristinsson J, Mala T. Abdominal pain and symptoms before and after roux-en-Y gastric bypass. BJS Open. 2019;**3**:317-326. DOI: 10.1002/bjs5.50148

[8] Peterli R, Wölnerhanssen BK, Peters T, Vetter D, Kröll D, Borbély Y, et al. Effect of laparoscopic sleeve gastrectomy vs laparoscopic roux-en-Y gastric bypass on weight loss in patients with morbid obesity: The SM-BOSS randomized clinical trial. Journal of the American Medical Association. 2018;**319**:255-265. DOI: 10.1001/jama.2017.20897

[9] Amor IB, Kassir R, Petrucciani N, Almunifi A, Debs T, Gugenheim J. An alternative technique of reversal of roux-en-Y gastric bypass: The small bowel limb transposition. Obesity Surgery. 2019;**29**:4142-4143. DOI: 10.1007/s11695-019-04158-y

[10] Wijngaarden LH, van Veldhuisen SL, Klaassen RA, van der Harst E, van Rossem CC, Demirkiran A, et al. Predicting symptom relief after reoperation for suspected internal herniation after laparoscopic roux-en-Y gastric bypass. Obesity Surgery. 2018;**28**:3801-3808. DOI: 10.1007/s11695-018-3404-8

[11] Alexandrou A, Sakarellos P, Davakis S, Vailas M, Dimitriou N, Papalampros A, et al. Revision of roux-en-Y gastric bypass for inadequate weight loss or weight regain. In Vivo. 2022;**36**:30-39. DOI: 10.21873/invivo.12673

[12] Plitzko G, Schmutz G, Kröll D, Nett PC, Borbély Y. Ulcer disease in the excluded segments after roux-en-Y gastric bypass: A current review of the literature. Obesity Surgery. 2021;**31**:1280-1289. DOI: 10.1007/s11695-020-05123-w

[13] Eriksen F, Carlsson ER, Munk JK, Madsbad S, Fenger M. Fractionated free fatty acids and their relation to diabetes status after roux-en-Y gastric bypass: A cohort study. Physiological Reports. 2021;**9**:e14708. DOI: 10.14814/phy2.14708

[14] Nuytens F, D'Hondt M, Van Rooy F, Vansteenkiste F, Pottel H, Abasbassi M, et al. Closure of mesenteric defects is associated with a higher incidence of small bowel obstruction due to adhesions after laparoscopic antecolic roux-en-y gastric bypass: A retrospective cohort study. International Journal of Surgery. 2019;**71**:149-155. DOI: 10.1016/j.ijsu.2019.09.017

[15] Zhang C, Zhang J, Zhou Z. Changes in fasting bile acid profiles after roux-en-Y gastric bypass and sleeve gastrectomy. Medicine (Baltimore). 2021;**100**:e23939. DOI: 10.1097/md.0000000000023939

[16] Chen GL, Kubat E, Eisenberg D. Prevalence of anemia 10 years after roux-en-Y gastric bypass in a single veterans affairs medical center. JAMA Surgery. 2018;**153**:86-87. DOI: 10.1001/jamasurg.2017.3158

[17] Laparoscopic sleeve gastrectomy. [Internet]. 2020. DOI: 10.1002/aorn.13309. Available from: https://aornjournal.onlinelibrary.wiley.com/ [Accessed: 06, Sept 2022]

[18] Garofalo F, Pescarus R, Denis R, Atlas H, Garneau P, Philie M, et al. Laparoscopic sleeve gastrectomy: A radiological guide to common postsurgical failure. Canadian Association of Radiologists Journal. 2018;**69**:184-196. DOI: 10.1016/j.carj.2017.10.004

[19] Batman B, Altun H. Benefits of suture reinforcement in laparoscopic sleeve gastrectomy. Surgical Laparoscopy, Endoscopy & Percutaneous Techniques. 2019;**29**:539-542. DOI: 10.1097/sle.0000000000000722

[20] Eckhouse SR. Comments on: Differences in the effect of laparoscopic sleeve gastrectomy and laparoscopic roux-en-Y gastric bypass on gut hormones: Systemic and meta-analysis. Surgery for Obesity and Related Diseases. 2021;**17**:e15-ee6. DOI: 10.1016/j.soard.2020.11.026

[21] Wang H, Lu J, Feng J, Wang Z. Staple line oversewing during laparoscopic sleeve gastrectomy. Annals of the Royal College of Surgeons of England. 2017;**99**:509-514. DOI: 10.1308/rcsann.2017.0074

[22] Saliba C, Nicolas G, Diab S, Joudi I, Tayar C. Gastrobronchial fistula following a laparoscopic sleeve gastrectomy. The American Journal of Case Reports. 2019;**20**:31-35. DOI: 10.12659/ajcr.910596

[23] Palermo M, Serra E. Laparoscopic sleeve gastrectomy: How do I do it. Journal of Laparoendoscopic & Advanced Surgical Techniques. Part A. 2020;**30**:2-5. DOI: 10.1089/lap.2019.0452

[24] Leca BM, Khan U, Abraham J, Halder L, Shuttlewood E, Shah N, et al. Laparoscopic adjustable gastric banding-should a second chance Be given? Obesity Surgery. 2020;**30**:2913-2919. DOI: 10.1007/s11695-020-04613-1

[25] Furbetta N, Cervelli R, Furbetta F. Laparoscopic adjustable gastric banding, the past, the present and the future. Annals of Translational Medicine. 2020;**8**:S4. DOI: 10.21037/atm.2019.09.17

[26] Li L, Yu H, Liang J, Guo Y, Peng S, Luo Y, et al. Meta-analysis of the effectiveness of laparoscopic adjustable

gastric banding versus laparoscopic sleeve gastrectomy for obesity. Medicine (Baltimore). 2019;**98**:e14735. DOI: 10.1097/md.0000000000014735

[27] Özden S, Saylam B, Avşar FM. Long-term results of the patients who were applied laparoscopic adjustable gastric banding. Turkish Journal of Surgery. 2019;**35**:79-85. DOI: 10.5578/turkjsurg.4038

[28] Mansour S, Borzellino G, Kluger Y, Khuri S. Unexpected gastrointestinal tract injury years following laparoscopic adjustable gastric banding. International Journal of Surgery Case Reports. 2020;**77**:412-417. DOI: 10.1016/j.ijscr.2020.11.023

[29] Pérez-Pevida B, Trifu DS, Kamocka A, Álvarez HJ. Malnutrition secondary to gastrojejunal stricture after biliopancreatic diversion. International Journal of Surgery Case Reports. 2018;**44**:230-232. DOI: 10.1016/j.ijscr.2018.02.040

[30] Steenackers N, Brouwers E, Mertens A, Van Cleynenbreugel S, Lannoo M, Flamaing J, et al. Late complications of biliopancreatic diversion in an older patient: A case report. BMC Geriatrics. 2021;**21**:631. DOI: 10.1186/s12877-021-02578-z

[31] Bianchi A, Pagan-Pomar A, Jimenez-Segovia M, Martinez-Corcoles JA, Gonzalez-Argenté FX. Biliopancreatic diversion in the surgical treatment of morbid obesity: Long-term results and metabolic consequences. Obesity Surgery. 2020;**30**:4234-4242. DOI: 10.1007/s11695-020-04777-w

[32] Jovani M, Al Ghamdi S, Bejjani M, Gandour B, Khashab MA. Switching the switch: Endoscopic reversal of a biliopancreatic diversion. VideoGIE. 2021;**6**:464-467. DOI: 10.1016/j.vgie.2021.06.004

[33] Milani C, Duranti S, Bottacini F, Casey E, Turroni F, Mahony J, et al. The first microbial colonizers of the human gut: Composition, activities, and health implications of the infant gut microbiota. Microbiology and Molecular Biology Reviews. 2017;**81**:17-36. DOI: 10.1128/mmbr.00036-17

[34] Cuevas-Sierra A, Ramos-Lopez O, Riezu-Boj JI, Milagro FI, Martinez JA. Diet, gut microbiota, and obesity: Links with host genetics and epigenetics and potential applications. Advances in Nutrition. 2019;**10**:S17-s30. DOI: 10.1093/advances/nmy078

[35] Gomes AC, Hoffmann C, Mota JF. The human gut microbiota: Metabolism and perspective in obesity. Gut Microbes. 2018;**9**:308-325. DOI: 10.1080/19490976.2018.1465157

[36] Torres-Fuentes C, Schellekens H, Dinan TG, Cryan JF. The microbiota-gut-brain axis in obesity. The Lancet Gastroenterology & Hepatology. 2017;**2**:747-756. DOI: 10.1016/s2468-1253(17)30147-4

[37] Crovesy L, Masterson D, Rosado EL. Profile of the gut microbiota of adults with obesity: A systematic review. European Journal of Clinical Nutrition. 2020;**74**:1251-1262. DOI: 10.1038/s41430-020-0607-6

[38] Strandwitz P. Neurotransmitter modulation by the gut microbiota. Brain Research. 2018;**1693**:128-133. DOI: 10.1016/j.brainres.2018.03.015

[39] Sánchez-Alcoholado L, Gutiérrez-Repiso C, Gómez-Pérez AM, García-Fuentes E, Tinahones FJ, Moreno-Indias I. Gut microbiota

adaptation after weight loss by roux-en-Y gastric bypass or sleeve gastrectomy bariatric surgeries. Surgery for Obesity and Related Diseases. 2019;**15**:1888-1895. DOI: 10.1016/j.soard.2019.08.551

[40] Steinert RE, Rehman A, Souto Lima EJ, Agamennone V, Schuren FHJ, Gero D, et al. Roux-en-Y gastric bypass surgery changes fungal and bacterial microbiota in morbidly obese patients-a pilot study. PLoS One. 2020;**15**:e0236936. DOI: 10.1371/journal.pone.0236936

[41] Faria SL, Santos A, Magro DO, Cazzo E, Assalin HB, Guadagnini D, et al. Gut microbiota modifications and weight regain in morbidly obese women after roux-en-Y gastric bypass. Obesity Surgery. 2020;**30**:4958-4966. DOI: 10.1007/s11695-020-04956-9

[42] Zizmare L, Boyle CN, Buss S, Louis S, Kuebler L, Mulay K, et al. Roux-En-Y gastric bypass (RYGB) surgery during high liquid sucrose diet leads to gut microbiota-related systematic alterations. International Journal of Molecular Sciences. 2022;**23**:1126. DOI: 10.3390/ijms23031126

[43] Fouladi F, Carroll IM, Sharpton TJ, Bulik-Sullivan E, Heinberg L, Steffen KJ, et al. A microbial signature following bariatric surgery is robustly consistent across multiple cohorts. Gut Microbes. 2021;**13**:1930872. DOI: 10.1080/19490976.2021.1930872

[44] Al Assal K, Prifti E, Belda E, Sala P, Clément K, Dao MC, et al. Gut microbiota profile of obese diabetic women submitted to roux-en-Y gastric bypass and its association with food intake and postoperative diabetes remission. Nutrients. 2020;**12**:278. DOI: 10.3390/nu12020278

[45] Liu Z, Coales I, Penney N, McDonald JAK, Phetcharaburanin J, Seyfried F, et al. A subset of roux-en-Y gastric bypass bacterial consortium colonizes the gut of nonsurgical rats without inducing host-microbe metabolic changes. mSystems. 2020;**5**:e01047-20. DOI: 10.1128/mSystems.01047-20

[46] Chaudhari SN, Luo JN, Harris DA, Aliakbarian H, Yao L, Paik D, et al. A microbial metabolite remodels the gut-liver axis following bariatric surgery. Cell Host & Microbe. 2021;**29**:408-24.e7. DOI: 10.1016/j.chom.2020.12.004

[47] Kindel TL, Gould J. Comment on: Effects of sleeve gastrectomy on the composition and diurnal oscillation of gut microbiota related to the metabolic improvements. Surgery for Obesity and Related Diseases. 2018;**14**:739-740. DOI: 10.1016/j.soard.2018.03.020

[48] Ikeda T, Aida M, Yoshida Y, Matsumoto S, Tanaka M, Nakayama J, et al. Alteration in faecal bile acids, gut microbial composition and diversity after laparoscopic sleeve gastrectomy. The British Journal of Surgery. 2020;**107**:1673-1685. DOI: 10.1002/bjs.11654

[49] Farin W, Oñate FP, Plassais J, Bonny C, Beglinger C, Woelnerhanssen B, et al. Impact of laparoscopic roux-en-Y gastric bypass and sleeve gastrectomy on gut microbiota: A metagenomic comparative analysis. Surgery for Obesity and Related Diseases. 2020;**16**:852-862. DOI: 10.1016/j.soard.2020.03.014

[50] Lin BY, Lin WD, Huang CK, Hsin MC, Lin WY, Pryor AD. Changes of gut microbiota between different weight reduction programs. Surgery for Obesity and Related Diseases. 2019;**15**:749-758. DOI: 10.1016/j.soard.2019.01.026

[51] Barron M, Atkinson SN, Kirby J, Kindel T. Sleeve gastrectomy prevents hypertension associated with unique

shifts in the gut microbiome. Surgical Endoscopy. 2021;**35**:5461-5467. DOI: 10.1007/s00464-020-08036-y

[52] Anhê FF, Varin TV, Schertzer JD, Marette A. The gut microbiota as a mediator of metabolic benefits after bariatric surgery. Canadian Journal of Diabetes. 2017;**41**:439-447. DOI: 10.1016/j.jcjd.2017.02.002

[53] Ilhan ZE, DiBaise JK, Isern NG, Hoyt DW, Marcus AK, Kang DW, et al. Distinctive microbiomes and metabolites linked with weight loss after gastric bypass, but not gastric banding. Thc ISME Journal. 2017;**11**:2047-2058. DOI: 10.1038/ismej.2017.71

[54] Mukorako P, Lopez C, Baraboi ED, Roy MC, Plamondon J, Lemoine N, et al. Alterations of gut microbiota after biliopancreatic diversion with duodenal switch in Wistar rats. Obesity Surgery. 2019;**29**:2831-2842. DOI: 10.1007/s11695-019-03911-7

Chapter 2

Revisional Bariatric Surgery

Awadh Alqahtani and Mohammad Almayouf

Abstract

Metabolic surgery is considered a valuable tool in treating obesity compared to the non-surgical approach. Its effectiveness is evident in the form of weight loss, eliminating obesity-related comorbidities, and improving quality of life. Hence, the rate of metabolic surgery conducted worldwide has risen dramatically, parallel to the increasing rates of obesity. Unfortunately, there are drawbacks to metabolic surgeries. Weight regain/insufficient weight loss is feared by the patient and bariatric surgeon and can occur with nonadherence to a healthy lifestyle and dietary habits. Long-term complications related to metabolic surgery are possible following any metabolic surgery (e.g., chronic reflux, malnutrition, and fistula). Revisional surgery is the most effective approach to combat these drawbacks, and therefore a bariatric surgeon should be familiar with it. This chapter will discuss the indication of revisional surgery, the preoperative workup, the surgical techniques, and the outcome of revisional surgery. The chapter will focus on the most commonly performed metabolic surgery, that is, laparoscopic adjustable gastric band, laparoscopic sleeve gastrectomy, laparoscopic Roux-en-Y gastric bypass, and laparoscopic one anastomosis gastric bypass. By the end of this chapter, the reader will be able to: (1) Define metabolic surgery failure and indications of the revision. (2) Be able to approach the patient preoperatively and formulate a plan. (3) Be knowledgeable about the main operative steps. (4) Be aware of the predicted outcome of revisional surgery.

Keywords: revisional surgery, adjustable gastric band, sleeve gastrectomy, Roux-en-Y gastrectomy, one anastomosis gastric bypass, laparoscopy

1. Introduction

Obesity is now considered an epidemic worldwide and rising at an alarming rate. Not only does obesity increase the chance of developing debilitating comorbidities and affects the quality of life, but also has a major load on health systems and increases costs [1]. One of the most effective tools to tackle obesity is bariatric surgery. It showed remarkable and durable results compared to other means, such as lifestyle changes and intensive medical management [2]. Despite its effectiveness, due to the sedentary lifestyle and the availability of calorie-dense foods, in addition to other factors, weight regain or failure to lose is becoming more prevalent. Other issues of surgical intervention, in general, are the possible occurrence of surgery-related specific complications. Hence, revisional surgery is becoming more popular recently to address these inconveniences. This chapter will address the most common revisional bariatric surgeries practiced.

2. Revision of laparoscopic adjustable gastric band

The laparoscopic adjustable gastric band (LAGB) was introduced in the 1970s with a simple weight loss mechanism for restricting food intake [3]. Since its implementation in the surgical practice, LAGB has shown promising results and gained popularity [4–6]. One of its attractiveness is its reversibility and less-invasive nature than other metabolic procedures [7]. Despite these remarks, LAGB has fallen behind other metabolic procedures. In the most recent IFSO data, LAGB is the fourth most common procedure behind the laparoscopic sleeve gastrectomy (LSG), laparoscopic Roux-en-Y gastric bypass (RYGB), and the one anastomosis gastric bypass (OAGB).

2.1 Indication for revision

With the development of other types of metabolic surgery, the efficacy and results sustainability of LAGB was questioned [8–10]. Another reason for the LAGB decline is the nature of the procedure of inserting a foreign body. This can lead to various complications like band intolerance (slippage, reflux, and esophageal dilatation], port/tube complications (bowel obstruction and infection), or even band erosion through the stomach wall [11]. Hence, band removal is probably inevitable due to different indications. These indications for revision vary in the literature (**Table 1**).

2.2 Preoperative workup

Before the operation, interviewing the patient by the managing team is crucial to accomplish the desired goals. Symptoms of band intolerance should be carefully assessed, such as epigastric pain, dysphagia, and regurgitation. Band deflation should be considered preoperatively. All patients should undergo an upper contrast study to evaluate the anatomy, assess for reflux/hiatal hernia, and assess if there is neo-pouch development or any signs of band slippage. Band erosion symptoms can vary significantly from being asymptomatic to port infection. Esophagogastroduodenoscopy (EGD) is a valuable tool that should be used if there is any suspicion of band erosion or significant reflux disease [17]. **Figure 1** provides a suggested pathway for AGB management.

Author	Number of patients	Band intolerance	Reflux	Band failure	Port/tube complications	Erosion
Emous et al. [12]	257	32.2%	NA	64.2%	0.5%	5.4%
Yeung et al. [13]	104	14%	12%	71%	3%	NA
Falk et al. [14]	211	60%	4.9%	20.5%	4.9%	4.3%
Jaber et al. [15]	85	63.5%	NA	22.4%	NA	1.2%
Kirshtein et al. [16]	214	61.6%	NA	9.8%	7%	13.1%

Table 1.
Indications of laparoscopic adjustable gastric band revision in selected studies.

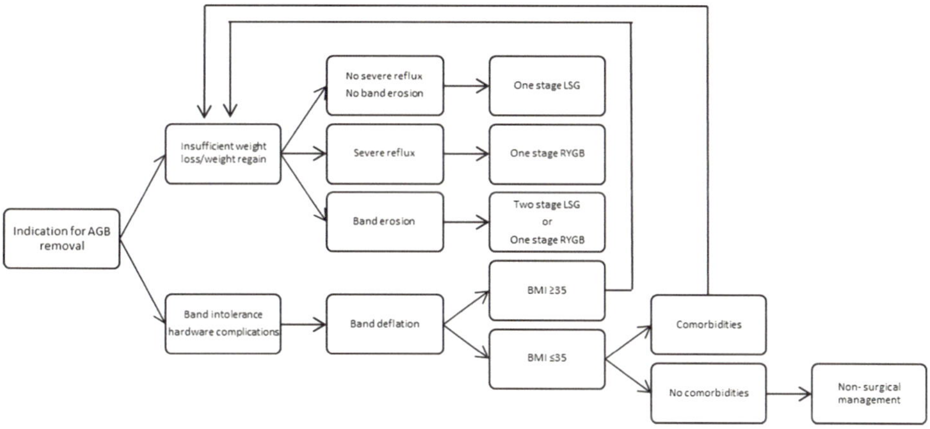

Figure 1.
Suggested pathway decision for adjustable gastric band revision.

2.3 The operation

All patients should receive preoperative antibiotics and prophylaxis for the venous thromboembolic event (VTE). After anesthesia induction, the site of the port should be marked. The abdomen is accessed using a 5 mm visiport at the left upper quadrant 5 cm from the umbilicus. Another 5 mm port in the left upper quadrant is placed at a planned incision site for port removal. A superior epigastric incision is used for Nathanson's retractor to assist with left hepatic lobe retraction. A 12 mm port is placed 5 cm to the right and superior to the umbilicus. Another 5 mm port is placed in the right upper quadrant. The adhesions of the band should be dissected thoroughly, making sure not to injure the stomach. Complete circumferential dissection is needed to remove the band (**Figure 2**). Then the tube can be divided near its insertion into the band. It is advisable to separate any fibrous tissue adherent to the stomach wall to

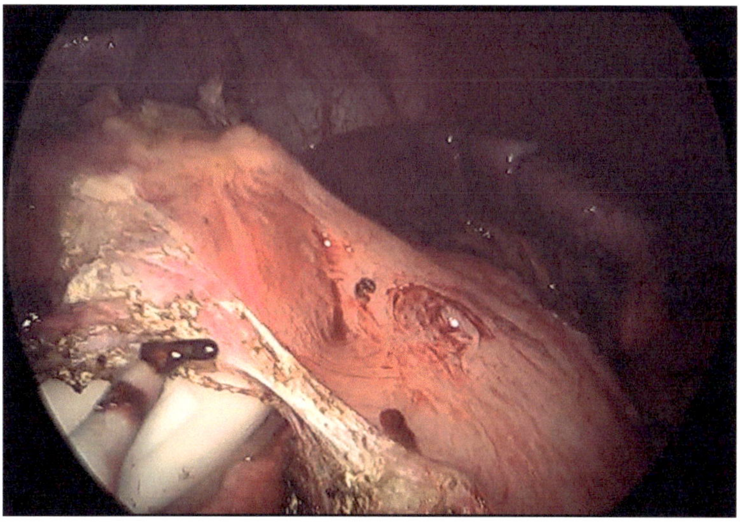

Figure 2.
Circumferential dissection around the band.

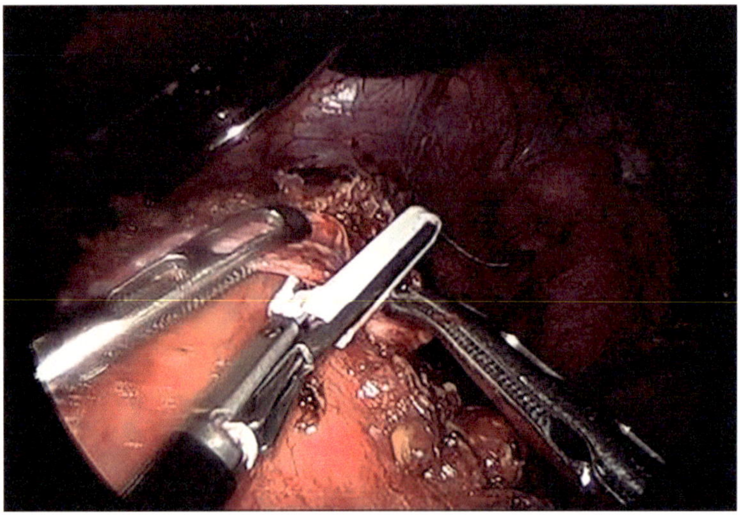

Figure 3.
Resection of fibrous tissue.

apply the stapler safely (**Figures 3** and **4**). Then laparoscopic sleeve gastrectomy is done by dividing the greater omentum to the gastroesophageal junction. It is crucial to assess for hiatal hernia. If present, complete mobilization of 2–3 cm intraabdominal esophagus should be accomplished with a posterior and anterior nonabsorbable suture repair (**Figures 5** and **6**). Creating the sleeve is started by applying staplers along a 36Fr bougie. We prefer to apply clips long the sleeve but not a full deployment to control bleeding. Reinforcement of the staple line with sutures is advisable. The procedure is completed by exteriorizing the band and the resected stomach, removing the port, and closing the skin.

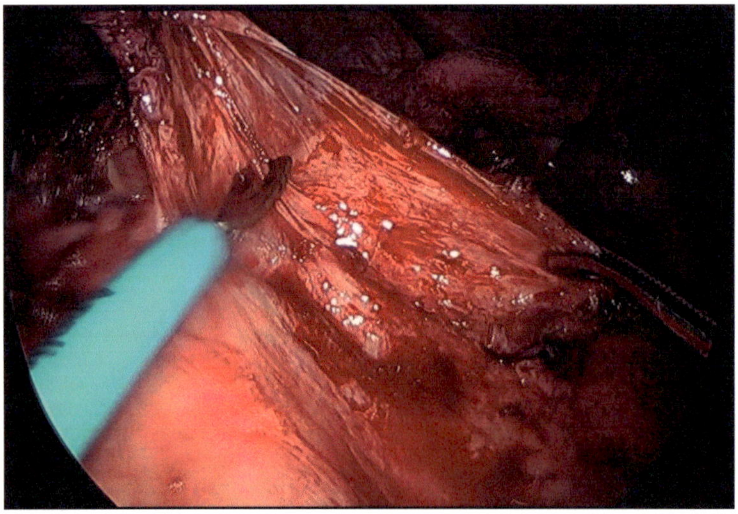

Figure 4.
Fine dissection of reactive tissue caused by the band before applying the stapler.

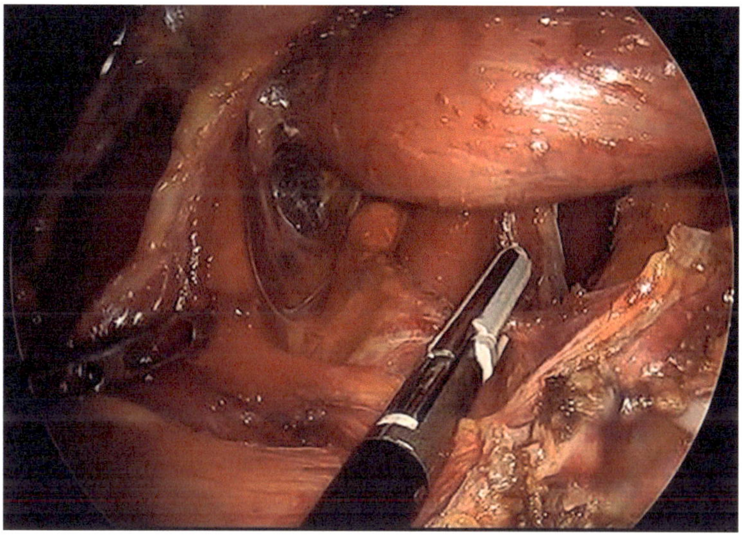

Figure 5.
Hiatal hernia dissection.

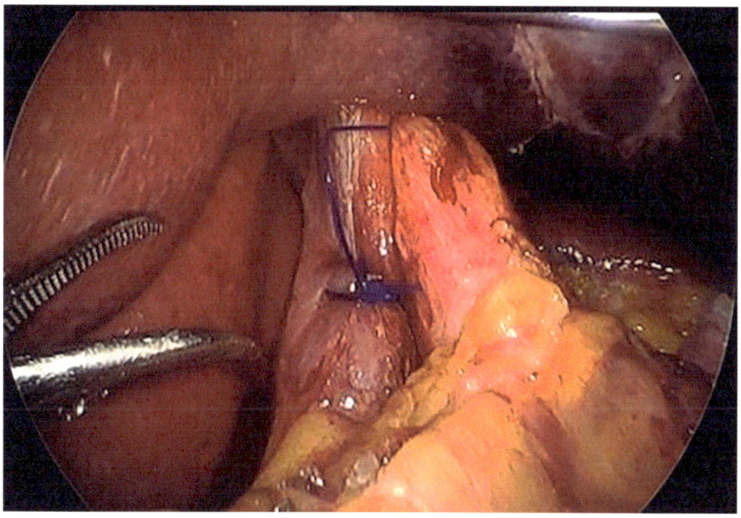

Figure 6.
Repaired hiatal hernia.

2.4 Postoperative care

Patients are encouraged to ambulate and use incentive spirometry. Intravenous fluid is kept until the next day, and the VTE prophylaxis is started 12 h from surgery. A contrast study is done to assess for any leaks or obstructions. If the contrast study is unremarkable, feeding with clear liquids is resumed. A clear discharge plan summarizing the diet program, medications, and follow-up appointments are described to the patient before leaving the hospital.

2.5 Outcome

As mentioned previously, revision of AGB is inevitable due to different indications. Even if the revision indication was band intolerance or slippage, removing the band only and not conducting another revisional surgery will likely lead to regaining weight. This observation was evident even in patients who follow a healthy diet and perform adequate exercises [16, 18]. Close follow-up for patients who underwent AGB removal and did not have weight regain/insufficient weight loss is crucial to prevent weight regain. There are diverse definitions of bariatric surgery failures from a weight loss perspective that can be used to indicate revision [19]. In the case of weight regain or insufficient weight loss, the type of revisional surgery is debated in the literature, with LSG and RYGB showing comparable results from excessive weight loss and resolution of comorbidities [20, 21]. Various factors can influence the decision on what kind of revision be conducted, including the patient's preference. Since LSG is undoubtfully less demanding from a technical point of view, we suggest choosing it as the revisional surgery for AGB as long as it is safe to be performed and there are no concerns of postoperative issues (severe reflux or band erosion). If severe reflux is evident by EGD (LA classification grade B/C) or band erosion was discovered preoperatively, the choice of RYGB is more appropriate than LSG. Performing the revision as one-stage versus two-stage is also an area of debate, especially with regards to anastomotic/staple line leak. Thickening of the stomach wall and the adherent capsule associated with the band are possible reasons behind the fear of performing the revision in one-stage. Staple line leak rate in one stage revision to LSG ranged from 0 to 6% in selected reports [22–24]. As for revision to RYGB in one-stage, the anastomotic leak rate was around 1% [25, 26]. The decision of one-stage versus two-stage procedure should be taken carefully. A patient's medical background is an important determinant factor. The condition and healthiness of the stomach after band removal should be assessed judiciously. In case of the diseased stomach wall or band erosion, a two-stage procedure might be the safer option [27].

3. Revision of laparoscopic sleeve gastrectomy

Laparoscopic sleeve gastrectomy (LSG) became one of the most common procedures conducted worldwide to combat obesity. Initially, it was introduced as the first-stage of a management plan for highly morbid patients with obesity, where another bariatric surgery is planned after weight loss [28]. Since it is increasing in popularity, an international expert panel consensus was introduced to clarify the indications and standardize the technique. The efficacy of LSG compared to other procedures was evident in the literature on weight loss and treating obesity-related diseases [29, 30]. Recently, the literature began to evaluate the long-term effectiveness (>10 years) of LSG, and it showed promising results [31]. With its relative ease compared to other bariatric surgery and the excellent outcomes, LSG became the most common bariatric procedure conducted worldwide. The exploding number of LSGs conducted will undoubtedly lead to an increased revision rate due to complications or weight loss issues, which are becoming more prevalent in the surgical practice.

3.1 Indication of revision

The failure of LSG from a weight-loss standpoint is multifactorial, including the technique implemented, lifestyle behaviors, and possible sleeve dilatation. The rate

Author	Number of patients	Weight regain/insufficient weight loss	Reflux	Weight regain/insufficient weight loss + reflux	others
Chang et al. [35]	69	28%	68%	0	10%
Poghosyan et al. [36]	72	100%	0	0	0
Mandeville et al. [37]	26	73.1%	7.7%	7.7%	0
Gadiot et al. [38]	44	86.3%	13.6%	0	0
Felsenreich et al. [39]	33	65.6%	34.3%	0	0

Table 2.
Indication of laparoscopic sleeve gastrectomy revision in selected studies.

of weight regain ranges from 530% [32]. Those who gained weight after an effective restrictive procedure will benefit from the addition of a malabsorptive feature. Reflux disease is a theoretical consequence of LSG. Since the stomach's lumen decreases in size following the procedure, intraluminal pressure increases, leading to a higher chance of gastric secretions backflow to the esophagus [33]. This phenomenon translates to what is known as de novo reflux disease, and it can be significant to the extent of intolerability affecting a patient's quality of life. Following LSG, the chance of hiatal hernia development is noteworthy and can potentiate reflux, which needs to be ruled out by EGD [34]. If the fundus is not resected while conducting LSG, it can also be a culprit in post LSG reflux disease, which an upper contrast study or EGD can discover (**Table 2**) [40]. In case of a twist or a stricture of the sleeve that is not amenable to stent or dilation, conversion to bypass is the best option (**Figure 7**).

3.2 Preoperative workup

It is essential to evaluate the pre-LSG weight and how much weight was lost during the patient's interview. Evaluating a patient's perspective about the reasons for bariatric surgery failure is crucial. If bad dietary habits were the main reason, consulting a dietician for education will help lose weight and maintain the loss after revisional surgery.

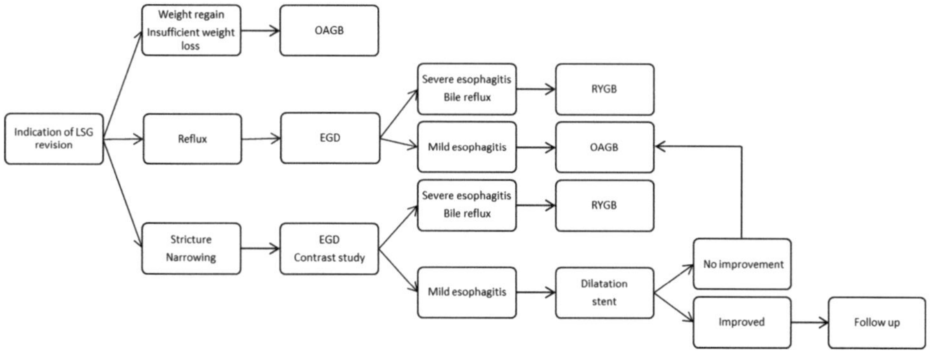

Figure 7.
Suggested pathway decision for sleeve gastrectomy revision.

All patients should undergo an upper GI contrast study to evaluate the status of the sleeve, if dilatation is present, remnant fundus or if there is a twist. Reflux symptoms (heartburn, frequent cough/choking, and using proton pump inhibitors) will require EGD. If there is a consequence of the reflux in the form of esophagitis, then offering RYGB is a safe option. In case of hiatal hernia discovery that can explain the reflux, OAGB can be offered but with a risk of reflux up to 30% in the postoperative period. If the patient is eligible for OAGB, it is essential to mention that reflux can occur after OAGB that can be controlled by avoiding reflux aggravators (large meals, spicy foods, and lying down after meals) and healthy eating habits. In case of biliary reflux, the safest option is RYGB. **Figure 5** provides a suggested management plan for the revision of LSG.

3.3 The operation

Preoperative preparations are followed similar to the previous section. After safe entry to the abdomen, we start counting the bowel, first starting from the duodenojejunal junction. If the patient's BMI is less than 40 kg/m^2, 150 cm of the bowel is bypassed. If the BMI is more than 40 kg/m^2, 180 cm of the bowel is bypassed. That point is labeled with clips. Adhesions are released from the area of previous stapling till the GEJ. The assessment for any hiatal hernia is critical. Repair of hiatal hernia is accomplished by anterior and posterior nonabsorbable monofilament sutures. At the incisura and below the crow's feet, we recommend the horizontal transection of the stomach with the highest stapling available (i.e., black reload) (**Figure 8**). A 36F bougie is introduced, and the pouch should be resized when applicable, avoiding narrowing the lumen (**Figure 9**). In preparation for the anastomosis, an enterotomy and gastrotomy are made. The gastrotomy should be made at the posterior aspect of the stomach to prevent bile reflux (**Figure 10**). An ante-colic gastrojejunostomy is constructed by a stapler fired at the 3 cm point joining the two lumens, then closing the defect with a 3-0 continuous absorbable suture in a double layer fashion (**Figure 11**). We highly recommend fixing the gastric pouch by omentopexy. Alignment stitches should be utilized to align and fix the anastomosis to prevent any kink or twist.

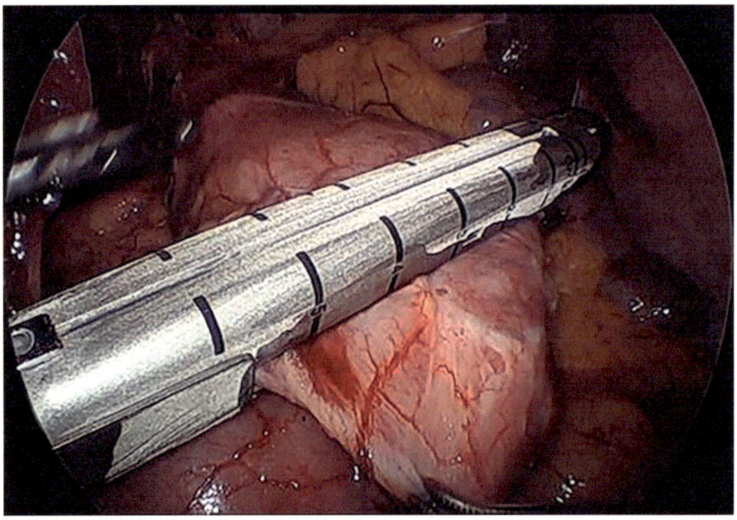

Figure 8.
Horizontal division of the sleeved stomach.

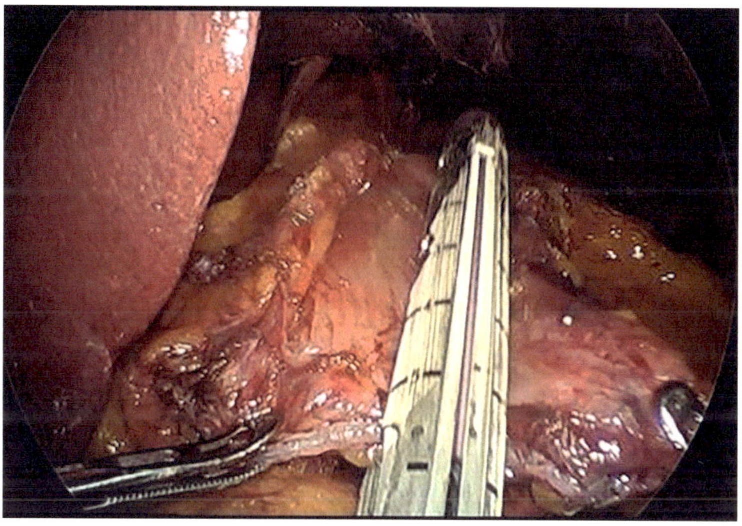

Figure 9.
Resizing the gastric pouch under the guidance of 36Fr bougie.

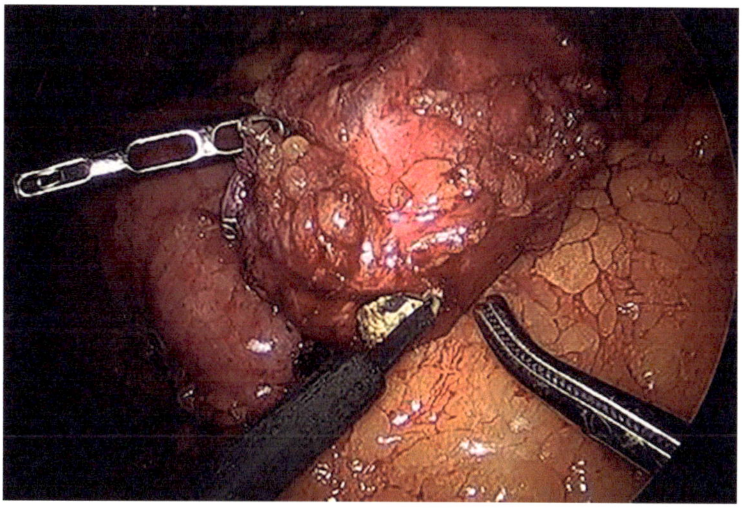

Figure 10.
A gastrotomy is made at the posterior aspect of the gastric pouch.

If the decision is to convert to RYGB, we highly recommend counting the whole bowel first. After forming the gastric pouch, a 120 cm alimentary limb is anastomosed to the pouch with a gastrojejunostomy technique similar to what was mentioned previously. A side-to-side jejunojejunostomy is made with 80–100 cm biliopancreatic limb. It is vital to allow an adequate common channel length to lower the risk of malabsorption. All mesenteric defects must be closed to prevent internal hernias. In case of a twist or stricture, and the decision to go for a bypass, it is important to make the GJ anastomosis above the stricture because the blood supply to that segment might be insufficient, which might threaten the anastomosis viability (**Figures 12** and **13**).

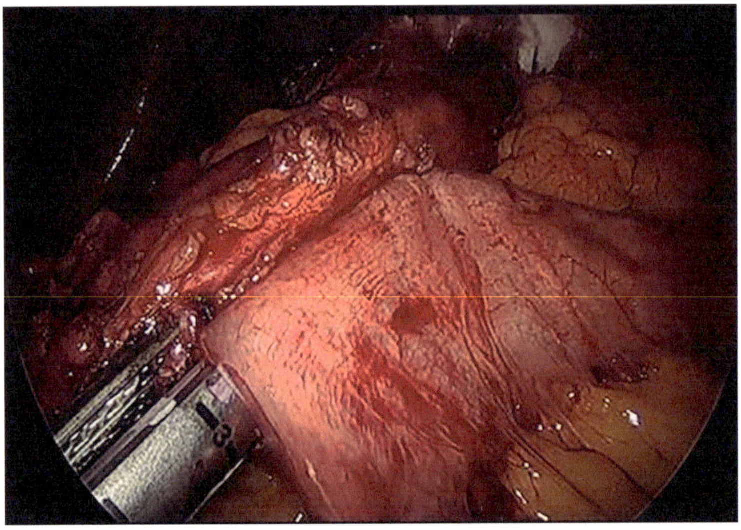

Figure 11.
A gastrojejunostomy is constructed at the 30 mm mark using a 60 mm stapler.

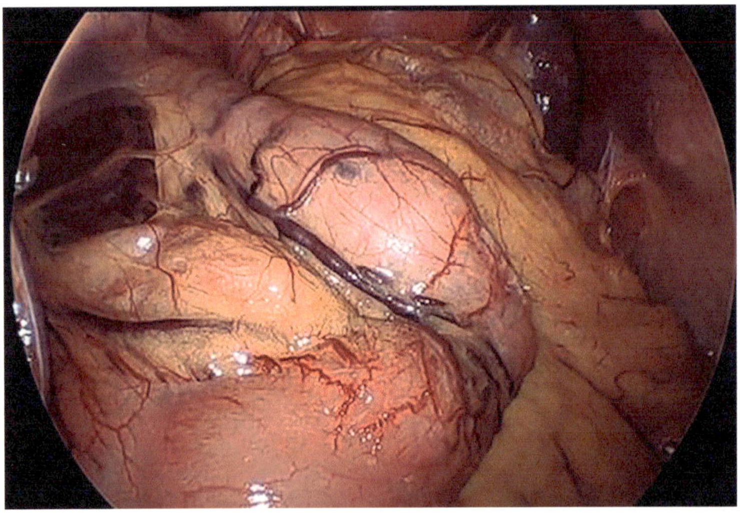

Figure 12.
Twist of the stomach after sleeve gastrectomy.

3.4 Postoperative care

Intravenous fluid should be kept on the first day until the upper GI study confirms free-flowing contrast through the anastomosis, with no interruption or delay of the flow. This is critical, especially after concomitant hiatal hernia repair. Ambulation and incentive spirometry use are necessary to be reminded by the managing team. Anticoagulant medications should be resumed based on the guidelines followed. Before discharge, instructions about diet progression, activity, and specific ominous symptoms requiring attention are explained to the patient.

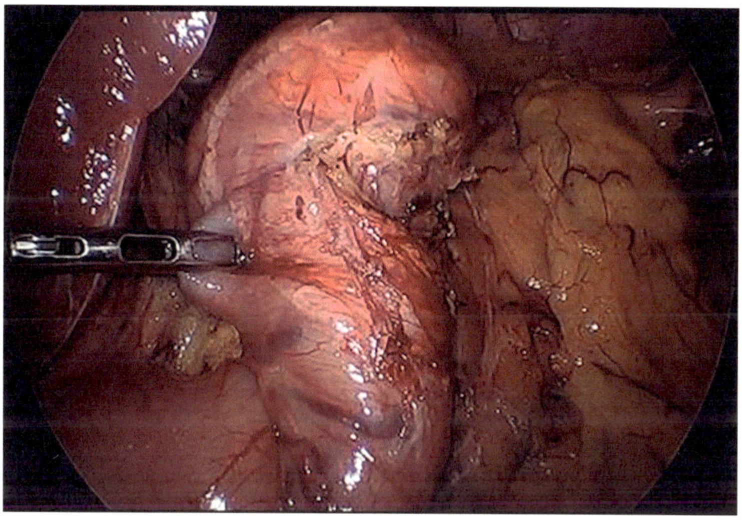

Figure 13.
Twisted sleeve. The dashed line illustrates the unequal stapling.

3.5 Outcome

The success of LSG in weight loss depends on several factors. Some are related to the technique conducted, like the size of the bougie used and the distance from the pylorus where the first stapler is applied [41]. Restricting oral intake is not only the reason for weight loss, but also LSG affects the hormones of interest involved in weight and hunger. The ghrelin level drops significantly postoperatively by removing the fundus, and the peptide YY (PYY) gets considerable elevation after the surgery. This observation probably explains the rapid satiety and hunger reduction during the early years after LSG [42]. Following dietary instructions and avoiding a sedentary lifestyle are key components of success [43]. As long as the procedure is done properly, predictors of weight regain/insufficient weight loss following LSG can be related mainly to dietary misbehavior and nonadherence to instructions [44]. Since restriction has failed in patients with WR/IWL following LSG, a rational strategy is adding a malabsorptive element in the surgical management. The classic revision of LSG is to convert to RYGB, but the OAGB seems to be a strong contender for two main reasons (**Table 3**). First, OAGB showed a comparative efficacy to RYGB as a rescue procedure, with less operative time and fewer complications [49]. Second, more options for managing weight recidivism can be achieved by adding a procedure before RYGB, which is the OAGB. In case OAGB fails, it can be converted smoothly to RYGB.

There are critiques mentioned in the literature expressing the disapproval of OAGB in some aspects. One of these remarks is the fear of bile reflux and the subsequent continuous esophageal irritation, which is worrisome. This is possible if the gastric pouch is short, increasing the chance of bile backflow to the stomach and ultimately in the esophagus. Keeping the gastric pouch long is critical to prevent the feared bile reflux, and being liberal in using “alignment stitches” or the so called “anti-reflux stitches” to prevent kinks or twists are critical elements in the procedure (**Figure 10**) [50, 51]. After improving the technique of the OAGB procedure, the rate of bile reflux following OAGB is reported to be around 0.7–2% [52, 53].

Author	Number of patients	Indication of revision	Time until revision (years)	Follow-up rate	Excessive weight loss	Length of BPL
Poghosyan et al [36]	72	IWL WR	NA	65% (5 year)	60% (1 year)	150, 200 cm
Gregs et al [45]	28	IWL 53% WR 46%	2 years	100% (1 year)	79% (1 year)	200 cm
Pizza et al [46]	59	IWL 20% WR 79%	2 years	NA	69%	200– 220 cm
Poublon et al [47]	65	IWL 30% WR 56%	NA	83% (1 year)	NA	180 cm
Rayman et al [48]	144	IWL 79% WR 20%	5 years	NA	58%	NA

Table 3.
Outcome following revision of sleeve gastrectomy to one anastomosis gastric bypass.

A large portion of the bariatric community classifies OAGB as a malabsorptive procedure. Malnutrition became an issue because the bypassed BPL can be as long as 300 cm in some practices. Reports showed severe nutritional deficiencies, hypoalbuminemia, and liver failure [54, 55]. In a survey conducted targeting IFSO members, all revisions due to malnutrition occurred when the BPL was 200 cm or more [56]. Because of OAGB's simplicity, the length of BPL is the only possible reason for this outcome. It seems that elongating the BPL is not beneficial from a weight-loss standpoint and endangers the patient with malnutrition and its dreadful consequences. Recently, it has been highly recommended not to exceed 180 cm of BPL length in order to prevent malnutrition, and at the same time, this limit will not compromise weight loss [55, 57].

The rate of reported GERD development after LSG ranged from 7.8 to 20%. It could be the consequence of fibers/ligaments division near the gastroesophageal junction, which alters and nullifies the angle of his features in protecting from reflux. Other factors include increased pressure because of the lumen narrowing or missing a hiatal hernia [58]. Unfortunately, when reflux develops after LSG due to a hiatal hernia, simply repairing the hiatal hernia showed disappointing results [59]. The applicability of OAGB in the treatment of reflux is a valid option in certain situations. If there is no severe reflux or Barret's esophagus on endoscopy, OAGB is a suitable option [60]. Clear communication with the patient about the possible recurrence of manageable reflux postoperatively is necessary.

4. Revision of Roux-en-Y gastric bypass

Since several decades ago, laparoscopic Roux-en-Y gastric bypass (RYGB) is still a valuable tool in the bariatric surgeon's arsenal. It has a unique configuration where it implements a restrictive mechanism by dividing the stomach and forming a small gastric pouch. Secondly, RYGB involves bypassing some of the small bowels by constructing the Roux limb/alimentary limb delivering the food and a biliopancreatic limb delivering the pancreaticobiliary juices and meeting at the start of the common channel where most of the absorption takes place. (Wolfe) The length of each limb is variable, and there is no clear consensus about the perfect measurements. However, what is agreed on is the efficacy of RYGB in weight reduction by several other mechanisms, including changes in eating behavior, the favorable elevation of gut hormones (GLP1 and PPY), and likely beneficial changes in energy expenditure [61]. The efficacy of RYGB was pronounced in the literature. With effective and sustainable weight loss and resolution of comorbidities, it is regarded as one of the most effective procedures to combat obesity and obesity-related diseases [2, 62].

4.1 Indication of revision

Despite the effectiveness of RYGB, sadly, it is not immune to the possibility of revisions. The most typical indication of revision after RYGB is the weight regain. We cannot stress enough the importance of interviewing the patient and evaluating one of the most critical factors contributing to weight-regain: dietary habits and lifestyle. Other possible anatomical causes of weight regain need further evaluation. Additional indications for revisions are bile reflux, which can happen in the case of a short alimentary limb [63]. Patients can complain of GERD symptoms post-RYGB, and the presence of a hiatal hernia; a large gastric pouch producing acid can explain this presentation.

4.2 Preoperative workup

Binge eating and loss of self-control can be significant contributing factors to weight regain following bariatric surgery. This issue can be ameliorated with a behavioral therapist and a qualified dietician [64]. Other aspects contributing to weight regain that are related to surgical factors include the diameter of GJ anastomosis, a gastro-gastric (GG) fistula, or a dilated gastric pouch [65–67]. It is an excellent practice to start with an upper contrast study to evaluate the aforementioned anatomical features. If a suspicion of wide GJ anastomosis or a GG fistula is present, an EGD is recommended [68]. Preoperative nutritional assessment and vitamin level could be valuable (**Figure 14**).

4.3 The operation

The procedure starts with proper and secure patient positioning. Access to the abdomen is achieved using a visiport at 5 cm above and to the left of the umbilicus. Other ports and liver retractors are inserted in a controlled manner. Counting the

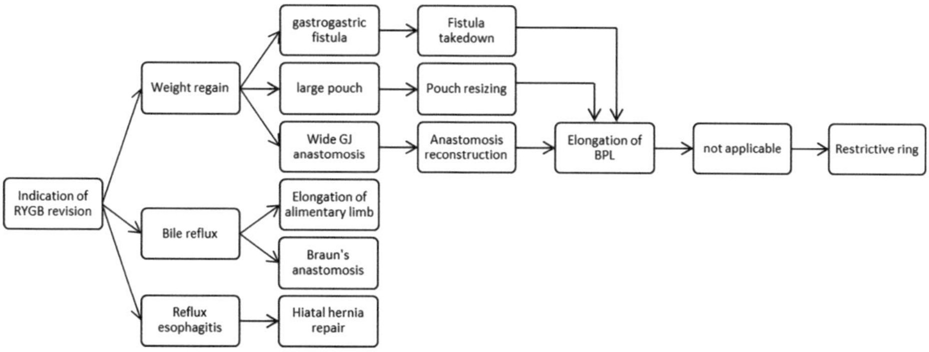

Figure 14.
Suggested pathway decision for revision of Roux-en-Y gastric bypass.

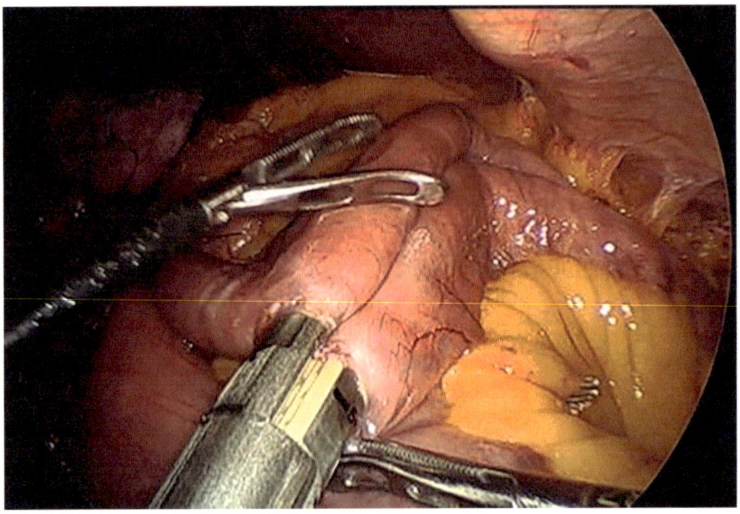

Figure 15.
Constructing a side-to-side jejunojejunostomy.

whole bowel at the beginning of the procedure and writing down the measurements is very helpful in formulating a plan. In case of weight regain, our practice dictates shortening the common channel to not less than five meters. The biliary limb is the one getting elongated. The jejunojejunostomy (JJ) will be divided at the distal end of the alimentary limb and brought down to the marked point of the new anastomosis. Enterotomies are made on the antimesenteric side, and a side-to-side anastomosis is made (**Figure 15**). Closure of the enterotomies is achieved using a double monofilament layer. The mesenteric defects need to be sought out and closed.

Resizing the gastric pouch when applicable is advantageous. In case of extensive adhesions near the gastrojejunostomy, we tend to avoid resizing the pouch if dissection is needed, which might jeopardize blood supply to the GJ anastomosis. It

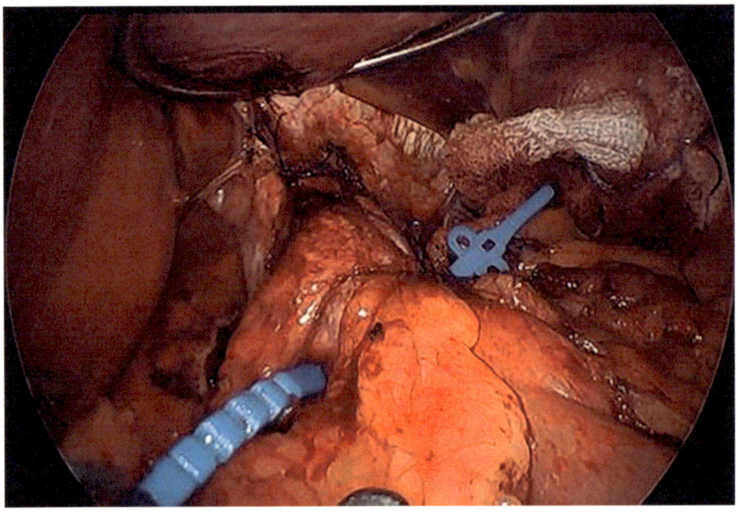

Figure 16.
A nonadjustable gastric band application around the gastric pouch above the gastrojejunostomy.

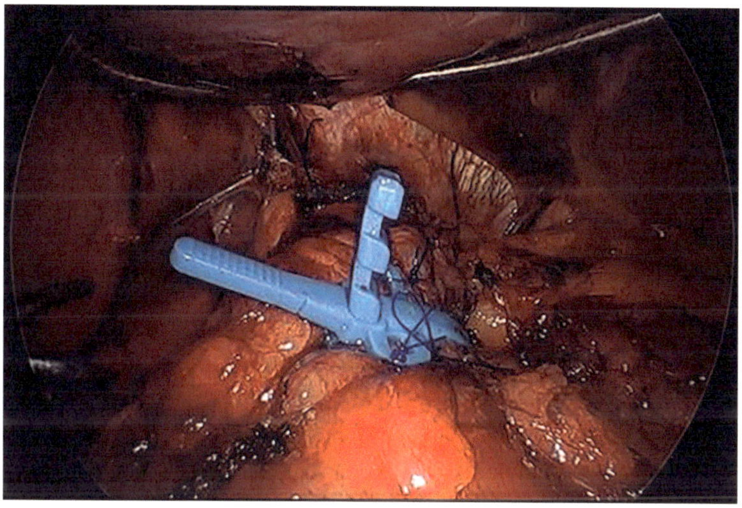

Figure 17.
A nonadjustable band is applied and sutured to the gastric pouch.

is essential to investigate the presence of hiatal hernia intra-operatively even if the preoperative scope did not show any signs of hiatal hernia. If present, the release of adhesions and mobilization of a 2–3 cm intrabdominal esophagus is needed. The hernia is closed using an anterior and posterior monofilament sutures. If the common channel is short and does not allow for JJ distalization, applying a nonadjustable restrictive ring might be applicable. Careful dissection proximal to the GJ anastomosis is needed, and it should be snugly applied with no constriction (**Figures 16** and **17**).

4.4 Postoperative care

According to the protocol, we tend to delay oral intake until oral contrast assures normal flowing contrast with no delays or leakage. After that, clear liquids can be started. Ambulation and respiratory exercise are crucial. Resumption of anticoagulants is started around 12 h after surgery and continued for 2–3 weeks after surgery. Instructions and education before discharge are given, with follow-up appointments and contact numbers in case of emergency.

4.5 Outcome

Since its introduction, RYGB has helped patients with obesity to lose weight and control their comorbidities. Changes in eating habits, food preferences, and hormonal changes are some of the mechanisms explaining the procedure's efficacy [69]. Although less technically demanding procedures are available, RYGB is still considered the preferable procedure in some areas worldwide. Several reports demonstrated the efficacy of RYGB and its durability from a weight-loss standpoint over 10 years, with a total weight reduction of >25% in 61–71% of patients [70–72]. Despite that, weight regain can happen regardless of the type of weight-reducing surgery. Around 30% of patients with obesity subjected to LRYGB had weight regain, and the cause seems multifactorial, including patient-related causes (binge eating and sedentary lifestyle) and elapsed time since surgery [73, 74].

Different approaches can be employed when revising the RYGB after weight-regain or insufficient weight loss. These include modification of bowel length, resizing the gastric pouch, applying a restrictive band, or a combination of these interventions.

4.5.1 Bowel length adjustments

Shortening the common channel to augment the malabsorptive component of RYGB is an intuitive option. Since the configuration of RYGB results in a different type of bowel based on what they deliver, two options arise that leads to shortening the common channel. Firstly, is elongating the Roux limb that ends with shortening of the common channel, and the biliary limb is not affected [75]. Although excess weight loss was excellent with this technique, the risk of nutritional deficiency and protein malabsorption was frequent [76]. The second option is elongating the biliary limb by shortening the common channel [77, 78]. This results in less but effective weight loss, with less risk of malnutrition. There is no consensus on which procedure is optimal, and both procedures are adequate. However, what is essential is to avoid detrimental nutritional deficiency and malnutrition. This can be achieved by measuring the bowel length and ensuring adequate bowel length for nutrient absorption. A total alimentary limb (the sum of Roux limb and common channel) of more than four to five meters is adequate to avoid malnutrition [79].

4.5.2 Resizing the gastric pouch only

Focusing on enhancing the restrictive part of RYGB seems a safe and valid decision for the management of weight regain. The option includes either stapling the gastric pouch, the GJ anastomosis or both, to reduce the volume [80]. The other method is the plication of the gastric pouch under the guidance of a bougie [81]. It is crucial to evaluate the effect of remnant candy cane that might increase the volume of the oral intake. Resizing the gastric pouch not only augments the restrictive nature of RYGB but also reduces GERD by eliminating more of the acid-producing cells [82].

4.5.3 Application of restrictive band

Bad eating habits can ensue after RYGB, probably due to the direct flow of food to the bowel. The size of the GJ anastomosis could be implicated in this phenomenon. Applying a band around the gastric pouch can prevent this hyperphagia through a simple restriction. Both types of band, that is, adjustable and nonadjustable, were examined and showed varying degrees of weight loss. In our opinion, band application seems less attractive compared to the remaining options because of the possible band complications (erosion and slippage) [83, 84].

Other available options include endoluminal revision, which has the lowest weight reduction compared to the other means [85, 86]. A combination of the options mentioned above is potentially valuable to maximize the chance of weight reduction. Careful patient selection and patient commitment are crucial to success.

5. Patient's compliance

Resolving obesity can be achieved by constructing a management plan between the surgeon and the patient. This plan includes several elements: the surgery, the follow-up appointments, and compliance with the instructions. These elements collectively contribute to weight loss and sustain the loss most of the time. Unfortunately, some patients fail to follow the plan recommended and end up with weight regain. Patients compliant with the follow-up appointment have better outcomes and more sustainability of weight loss. This is true because the surgeon can keep up with the patient's progress, catch any derails from the management plan, and correct any mistakes that might hinder achieving the goals [87].

The managing team should seek the possibility of the patient's noncompliance during the preoperative interview. Any indication of an eating disorder (binge eating and anorexia nervosa) should trigger a referral to a behavioral therapist before surgery. Patients with eating disorders have a high chance of failure if not addressed and managed preoperatively [88]. It is crucial to clarify to the patient that bariatric surgeries are a tool to help in weight loss with excellent efficacy. However, keeping a healthy lifestyle and good dietary habits is vital and should not be undermined.

6. Conclusion

Bariatric surgery is an effective tool to manage obesity, reverse obesity-related comorbidities, and improve quality of life. Weight regain or surgical complication following bariatric surgery is not uncommon. The appropriate approach for those patients who were unfortunate with their results should be thorough and systematic. A multidisciplinary team comprising the surgeon, an internist, a behavioral therapist, and a qualified dietician is highly recommended. These patients need complete investigation to assess their suitability for any potential surgical intervention. Patient participation in the management plan by following the instruction and changing lifestyle habits is crucial.

Author details

Awadh Alqahtani[1] and Mohammad Almayouf[2]*

1 Department of Surgery, King Saud University, College of Medicine, Riyadh, Saudi Arabia

2 Department of Surgery, Prince Sattam bin Abdulaziz University, College of Medicine, Alkharj, Saudi Arabia

*Address all correspondence to: mohammad.almayouf@outlook.com

References

[1] Smith KB, Smith MS. Obesity statistics. Primary Care: Clinics in Office Practice. 2016;**43**(1):121-135

[2] Schauer PR, Bhatt DL, Kirwan JP, Wolski K, Aminian A, Brethauer SA, et al. Bariatric surgery versus intensive medical therapy for diabetes—5-year outcomes. The New England Journal of Medicine. 2017;**376**:641-651

[3] Buchwald H. Introduction and current status of bariatric procedures. Surgery for Obesity and Related Diseases. 2008;**4**(3):S1-S6

[4] O'Brien PE, MacDonald L, Anderson M, Brennan L, Brown WA. Long-term outcomes after bariatric surgery: Fifteen-year follow-up of adjustable gastric banding and a systematic review of the bariatric surgical literature. Annals of Surgery. 2013;**257**(1):87-94

[5] O'Brien PE, Brennan L, Laurie C, Brown W. Intensive medical weight loss or laparoscopic adjustable gastric banding in the treatment of mild to moderate obesity: Long-term follow-up of a prospective randomised trial. Obesity Surgery. 2013;**23**(9):1345-1353

[6] Furbetta N, Gragnani F, Flauti G, Guidi F, Furbetta F. Laparoscopic adjustable gastric banding on 3566 patients up to 20-year follow-up: Long-term results of a standardized technique. Surgery for Obesity and Related Diseases. 2019;**15**(3):409-416

[7] Opozda M, Wittert G, Chur-Hansen A. Patients* reasons for and against undergoing Roux-en-Y gastric bypass, adjustable gastric banding, and vertical sleeve gastrectomy. Surgery for Obesity and Related Diseases. 2017;**13**(11):1887-1896

[8] Nguyen NT, Kim E, Vu S, Phelan M. Ten-year outcomes of a prospective randomized trial of laparoscopic gastric bypass versus laparoscopic gastric banding. Annals of Surgery. 2018;**268**(1):106

[9] Lee JH, Nguyen QN, Le QA. Comparative effectiveness of 3 bariatric surgery procedures: Roux-en-Y gastric bypass, laparoscopic adjustable gastric band, and sleeve gastrectomy. Surgery for Obesity and Related Diseases. 2016;**12**(5):997-1002

[10] Carlin AM, Zeni TM, English WJ, Hawasli AA, Genaw JA, Krause KR, et al. The comparative effectiveness of sleeve gastrectomy, gastric bypass, and adjustable gastric banding procedures for the treatment of morbid obesity. Annals of Surgery. 2013;**257**(5):791-797

[11] Shen X, Zhang X, Bi J, Yin K. Long-term complications requiring reoperations after laparoscopic adjustable gastric banding: A systematic review. Surgery for Obesity and Related Diseases. 2015;**11**(4):956-964

[12] Emous M, Apers J, Hoff C, Van Beek AP, Totté E. Conversion of failed laparoscopic adjustable gastric banding to Roux-en-Y gastric bypass is safe as a single-step procedure. Surgical Endoscopy. 2015;**29**(8):2217-2223

[13] Yeung L, Durkan B, Barrett A, Kraft C, Vu K, Phillips E, et al. Single-stage revision from gastric band to gastric bypass or sleeve gastrectomy: 6- and 12-month outcomes. Surgical Endoscopy. 2016;**30**(6):2244-2250

[14] Falk V, Sheppard C, Kanji A, Birch D, Karmali S, de Gara C. The fate of laparoscopic adjustable gastric band removal. Canadian Journal of Surgery. 2019;**62**(5):328

[15] Jaber J, Glenn J, Podkameni D, Soto F. A 5-year history of laparoscopic gastric band removals: An analysis of complications and associated comorbidities. Obesity Surgery. 2019;**29**(4):1202-1206

[16] Kirshtein B, Kirshtein A, Perry Z, Ovnat A, Lantsberg L, Avinoach E, et al. Laparoscopic adjustable gastric band removal and outcome of subsequent revisional bariatric procedures: A retrospective review of 214 consecutive patients. International Journal of Surgery. 2016;**27**:133-137

[17] Nocca D, Frering V, Gallix B, des Hons CD, Noël P, Foulonge MA, et al. Migration of adjustable gastric banding from a cohort study of 4236 patients. Surgical Endoscopy and other Interventional Techniques. 2005;**19**(7):947-950

[18] Aarts EO, Dogan K, Koehestanie P, Janssen IM, Berends FJ. What happens after gastric band removal without additional bariatric surgery. Surgery for Obesity and Related Diseases. 2014;**10**(6):1092-1096

[19] Mann JP, Jakes AD, Hayden JD, Barth JH. Systematic review of definitions of failure in revisional bariatric surgery. Obesity surgery. 2015 Mar;**25**(3):571-574

[20] Moon RC, Teixeira AF, Jawad MA. Conversion of failed laparoscopic adjustable gastric banding: sleeve gastrectomy or Roux-en-Y gastric bypass?. Surgery for Obesity and Related Diseases. 2013 Nov 1;**9**(6):901-907

[21] Angrisani L, Vitiello A, Santonicola A, Hasani A, De Luca M, Iovino P. Roux-en-Y gastric bypass versus sleeve gastrectomy as revisional procedures after adjustable gastric band: 5-year outcomes. Obesity Surgery. 2017 Jun;**27**(6):1430-1477

[22] Pencovich N, Lahat G, Goldray O, Abu-Abeid S, Klausner JM, Meron Eldar S. Safety and outcome of laparoscopic sleeve gastrectomy following removal of adjustable gastric banding: lessons from 109 patients in a single center and review of the literature. Obesity surgery. 2017 May;**27**(5):1266-1270

[23] Alqahtani AR, Elahmedi M, Alamri H, Mohammed R, Darwish F, Ahmed AM. Laparoscopic removal of poor outcome gastric banding with concomitant sleeve gastrectomy. Obesity surgery. 2013 Jun;**23**(6):782-787

[24] Acholonu E, McBean E, Bellorin O, Szomstein S, Rosenthal RJ. Safety and short-term outcomes of laparoscopic sleeve gastrectomy as a revisional approach for failed laparoscopic adjustable gastric banding in the treatment of morbid obesity. Obesity surgery. 2009 Dec;**19**(12):1612-1616

[25] Marin-Perez P, Betancourt A, Lamota M, Lo Menzo E, Szomstein S, Rosenthal R. Outcomes after laparoscopic conversion of failed adjustable gastric banding to sleeve gastrectomy or Roux-en-Y gastric bypass. Journal of British Surgery. 2014 Feb;**101**(3):254-260

[26] Aarts E, Koehestanie P, Dogan K, Berends F, Janssen I. Revisional surgery after failed gastric banding: results of one-stage conversion to RYGB in 195 patients. Surgery for Obesity and Related Diseases. 2014 Nov 1;**10**(6):1077-1083

[27] Super J, Charalampakis V, Tahrani AA, Kumar S, Bankenahally R, Raghuraman G, et al. Safety and feasibility of revisional bariatric surgery following Laparoscopic Adjustable Gastric Band–Outcomes from a large UK private practice. Obesity research & clinical practice. 2021 Jul 1;**15**(4):381-386

[28] Cottam D, Qureshi FG, Mattar SG, Sharma S, Holover S, Bonanomi G, et al. Laparoscopic sleeve gastrectomy as an initial weight-loss procedure for high-risk patients with morbid obesity. Surgical

Endoscopy and Other Interventional Techniques. 2006 Jun;**20**(6):859-863

[29] Trastulli S, Desiderio J, Guarino S, Cirocchi R, Scalercio V, Noya G, et al. Laparoscopic sleeve gastrectomy compared with other bariatric surgical procedures: a systematic review of randomized trials. Surgery for obesity and related diseases. 2013 Sep 1;**9**(5):816-829

[30] Shenoy SS, Gilliam A, Mehanna A, Kanakala V, Bussa G, Gill T, et al. Laparoscopic sleeve gastrectomy versus laparoscopic Roux-en-Y Gastric bypass in elderly bariatric patients: safety and efficacy—a systematic review and meta-analysis. Obesity surgery. 2020 Nov;**30**(11):4467-4473

[31] Kraljević M, Cordasco V, Schneider R, Peters T, Slawik M, Wölnerhanssen B, et al. Long-term effects of laparoscopic sleeve gastrectomy: what are the results beyond 10 years?. Obesity Surgery. 2021 Aug;**31**(8):3427-3433

[32] Lauti M, Kularatna M, Hill AG, MacCormick AD. Weight regain following sleeve gastrectomy—a systematic review. Obesity surgery. 2016 Jun;**26**(6):1326-1334

[33] Chern TY, Chan DL, Maani J, Ferguson JS, Talbot ML. High-resolution impedance manometry and 24-hour multichannel intraluminal impedance with pH testing before and after sleeve gastrectomy: de novo reflux in a prospective series. Surgery for Obesity and Related Diseases. 2021 Feb 1;**17**(2):329-337

[34] Saba J, Bravo M, Rivas E, Fernández R, Pérez-Castilla A, Zajjur J. Incidence of de novo hiatal hernia after laparoscopic sleeve gastrectomy. Obesity Surgery. 2020 Oct;**30**(10):3730-3734

[35] Chang DM, Lee WJ, Chen JC, Ser KH, Tsai PL, Lee YC. Thirteen-year experience of laparoscopic sleeve gastrectomy: Surgical risk, weight loss, and revision procedures. Obesity Surgery. 2018;**28**(10):2991-2997. Epub 2018/06/23. DOI: 10.1007/s11695-018-3344-3

[36] Poghosyan T, Alameh A, Bruzzi M, Faul A, Rives-Lange C, Zinzindohoue F, et al. Conversion of sleeve gastrectomy to one anastomosis gastric bypass for weight loss failure. Obesity Surgery. 2019;**29**(8):2436-2441. Epub 2019/04/05. DOI: 10.1007/s11695-019-03864-x

[37] Mandeville Y, Van Looveren R, Vancoillie PJ, Verbeke X, Vandendriessche K, Vuylsteke P, et al. Moderating the enthusiasm of sleeve gastrectomy: Up to fifty percent of reflux symptoms after ten years in a consecutive series of one hundred laparoscopic sleeve gastrectomies. Obesity Surgery. 2017;**27**(7):1797-1803. Epub 2017/02/13. DOI: 10.1007/s11695-017-2567-z

[38] Gadiot RPM, Biter LU, van Mil S, Zengerink HF, Apers J, Mannaerts GHH. Long-term results of laparoscopic sleeve gastrectomy for morbid obesity: 5 to 8-Year Results. Obesity Surgery. 2017;**27**(1):59-63. DOI: 10.1007/s11695-016-2235-8

[39] Felsenreich DM, Langer FB, Kefurt R, Panhofer P, Schermann M, Beckerhinn P, et al. Weight loss, weight regain, and conversions to Roux-en-Y gastric bypass: 10-year results of laparoscopic sleeve gastrectomy. Surgery for Obesity and Related Diseases. 2016;**12**(9):1655-1662. Epub 2016/06/19. DOI: 10.1016/j.soard.2016.02.021

[40] Daes J, Jimenez ME, Said N, Daza JC, Dennis R. Laparoscopic sleeve gastrectomy: symptoms of gastroesophageal reflux can be reduced by changes in surgical technique. Obesity surgery. 2012 Dec;**22**(12):1874-1879

[41] Abd Ellatif ME, Abdallah E, Askar W, Thabet W, Aboushady M, Abbas AE, et al. Long term predictors of success after laparoscopic sleeve gastrectomy. International journal of surgery. 2014 May 1;**12**(5):504-508

[42] Karamanakos SN, Vagenas K, Kalfarentzos F, Alexandrides TK. Weight loss, appetite suppression, and changes in fasting and postprandial ghrelin and peptide-YY levels after Roux-en-Y gastric bypass and sleeve gastrectomy: a prospective, double blind study. Annals of surgery. 2008 Mar 1;**247**(3):401-407

[43] Keren D, Matter I, Lavy A. Lifestyle modification parallels to sleeve success. Obesity surgery. 2014 May;**24**(5):735-740

[44] Yu Y, Klem ML, Kalarchian MA, Ji M, Burke LE. Predictors of weight regain after sleeve gastrectomy: an integrative review. Surgery for Obesity and Related Diseases. 2019 Jun 1;**15**(6):995-1005

[45] Gerges WB, Omran H, Makram F. Conversion of laparoscopic sleeve gastrectomy after weight loss failure into laparoscopic one anastomosis gastric bypass: short-term safety and efficacy and effect of indications on outcome. Surgical Endoscopy. 2022 Feb;**36**(2):1080-1089

[46] Pizza F, D'Antonio D, Carbonell Asins JA, Lucido FS, Tolone S, Docimo L, et al. One anastomosis gastric bypass after sleeve gastrectomy failure: Does a single procedure fit for all. Obesity Surgery. 2021;**31**(4):1722-1732. Epub 2021/01/05. DOI: 10.1007/s11695-020-05191-y

[47] Poublon N, Chidi I, Bethlehem M, Kuipers E, Gadiot R, Emous M, et al. One anastomosis gastric bypass vs. Roux-en-Y gastric bypass, remedy for insufficient weight loss and weight regain after failed restrictive bariatric surgery. Obesity Surgery. 2020;**30**(9):3287-3294. Epub 2020/04/21. DOI: 10.1007/s11695-020-04536-x

[48] Rayman S, Assaf D, Azran C, Sroka G, Assalia A, Beglaibter N, et al. Sleeve gastrectomy failure-revision to laparoscopic one-anastomosis gastric bypass or Roux-n-Y gastric bypass: A multicenter study. Obesity Surgery. 2021;**31**(7):2927-2934. Epub 2021/03/26. DOI: 10.1007/s11695-021-05334-9

[49] Chiappetta S, Stier C, Scheffel O, Squillante S, Weiner RA. Mini/one anastomosis gastric bypass versus Roux-en-Y gastric bypass as a second step procedure after sleeve gastrectomy—a retrospective cohort study. Obesity Surgery. 2019 Mar;**29**(3):819-827

[50] Luque-de-León E, Carbajo MA. Conversion of one-anastomosis gastric bypass (OAGB) is rarely needed if standard operative techniques are performed. Obesity surgery. 2016 Jul;**26**(7):1588-1591

[51] Musella M, Susa A, Manno E, De Luca M, Greco F, Raffaelli M, et al. Complications following the mini/one anastomosis gastric bypass (MGB/OAGB): A multi-institutional survey on 2678 patients with a mid-term (5 years) follow-up. Obesity Surgery. 2017;**27**(11):2956-2967. Epub 2017/06/02. DOI: 10.1007/s11695-017-2726-2

[52] Georgiadou D, Sergentanis TN, Nixon A, Diamantis T, Tsigris C, Psaltopoulou T. Efficacy and safety of laparoscopic mini gastric bypass. A systematic review. Surgery for obesity and related diseases. 2014 Sep 1;**10**(5):984-991

[53] Chevallier JM, Arman GA, Guenzi M, Rau C, Bruzzi M, Beaupel N, et al. One thousand single anastomosis (omega loop) gastric bypasses to treat morbid obesity in a 7-year period: outcomes show

few complications and good efficacy. Obesity surgery. 2015 Jun;**25**(6):951-958

[54] Khalaj A, Kalantar Motamedi MA, Mousapour P, Valizadeh M, Barzin M. Protein-calorie malnutrition requiring revisional surgery after one-anastomosis-mini-gastric bypass (OAGB-MGB): case series from the Tehran Obesity Treatment Study (TOTS). Obesity Surgery. 2019 Jun;**29**(6):1714-1720

[55] Ahuja A, Tantia O, Goyal G, Chaudhuri T, Khanna S, Poddar A, et al. MGB-OAGB: effect of biliopancreatic limb length on nutritional deficiency, weight loss, and comorbidity resolution. Obesity Surgery. 2018 Nov;**28**(11):3439-3445

[56] Haddad A, Bashir A, Fobi M, Higa K, Herrera MF, Torres AJ, et al. The IFSO worldwide one anastomosis gastric bypass survey: techniques and outcomes?. Obesity Surgery. 2021 Apr;**31**(4):1411-1421

[57] Boyle M, Mahawar K. One anastomosis gastric bypass performed with a 150-cm biliopancreatic limb delivers weight loss outcomes similar to those with a 200-cm biliopancreatic limb at 18-24 months. Obesity Surgery. 2020 Apr;**30**(4):1258-1264

[58] Melissas J, Braghetto I, Molina JC, Silecchia G, Iossa A, Iannelli A, et al. Gastroesophageal reflux disease and sleeve gastrectomy. Obesity Surgery. 2015;**25**(12):2430-2435. DOI: 10.1007/s11695-015-1906-1

[59] Soong T-C, Almalki OM, Lee W-J, Ser K-H, Chen J-C, Wu C-C, et al. Revision of sleeve gastrectomy with hiatal repair with gastropexy for gastroesophageal reflux disease. Obesity Surgery. 2019;**29**(8):2381-2386. DOI: 10.1007/s11695-019-03853-0

[60] Mahawar KK, Himpens J, Shikora SA, Chevallier J-M, Lakdawala M, De Luca M, et al. The first consensus statement on one anastomosis/mini gastric bypass (OAGB/MGB) using a modified delphi approach. Obesity Surgery. 2018;**28**(2):303-312. DOI: 10.1007/s11695-017-3070-2

[61] Lutz TA, Bueter M. The physiology underlying Roux-en-Y gastric bypass: A status report. American Journal of Physiology—Regulatory, Integrative and Comparative. 2014;**307**(11):R1275-R1291. Epub 2014/09/26. DOI: 10.1152/ajpregu.00185.2014

[62] Spivak H, Abdelmelek MF, Beltran OR, Ng AW, Kitahama S. Long-term outcomes of laparoscopic adjustable gastric banding and laparoscopic Roux-en-Y gastric bypass in the United States. Surgical Endoscopy. 2012;**26**(7):1909-1919. DOI: 10.1007/s00464-011-2125-z

[63] Boyle M, Mahawar K. One anastomosis gastric bypass performed with a 150-cm biliopancreatic limb delivers weight loss outcomes similar to those with a 200-cm biliopancreatic limb at 18-24 months. Obesity Surgery. 2020 Apr;**5**(1):27-30

[64] Kalarchian MA, Marcus MD, Wilson GT, Labouvie EW, Brolin RE, LaMarca LB. Binge eating among gastric bypass patients at long-term follow-up. Obesity Surgery. 2002 Apr;**12**(2):270-275

[65] Dayyeh BK, Lautz DB, Thompson CC. Gastrojejunal stoma diameter predicts weight regain after Roux-en-Y gastric bypass. Clinical Gastroenterology and Hepatology. 2011 Mar 1;**9**(3):228-233

[66] Carrodeguas L, Szomstein S, Soto F, Whipple O, Simpfendorfer C, Gonzalvo JP, et al. Management of gastrogastric fistulas after divided Roux-en-Y gastric bypass surgery for morbid obesity: analysis of 1292 consecutive patients and review of literature. Surgery for Obesity and Related Diseases. 2005 Sep 1;**1**(5):467-474

[67] Heneghan HM, Yimcharoen P, Brethauer SA, Kroh M, Chand B. Influence of pouch and stoma size on weight loss after gastric bypass. Surgery for Obesity and Related Diseases. 2012 Jul 1;**8**(4):408-415

[68] Brethauer SA, Nfonsam V, Sherman V, Udomsawaengsup S, Schauer PR, Chand B. Endoscopy and upper gastrointestinal contrast studies are complementary in evaluation of weight regain after bariatric surgery. Surgery for Obesity and Related Diseases. 2006 Nov 1;**2**(6):643-648

[69] Abdeen G, Le Roux CW. Mechanism underlying the weight loss and complications of Roux-en-Y gastric bypass. Review. Obesity surgery. 2016 Feb;**26**(2):410-421

[70] Guimarães M, Osório C, Silva D, Almeida RF, Reis A, Cardoso S, et al. How Sustained is Roux-en-Y Gastric Bypass Long-term Efficacy?. Obesity Surgery. 2021 Aug;**31**(8):3623-3629

[71] Gorecki P, McClelland PH, Kabata K, Khusid E, Zenilman ME. Weight loss dynamics following laparoscopic Roux-en-Y gastric bypass. An analysis of 10-year follow-up data. Surgical Endoscopy. 2021 Sep;**35**(9):5315-5321

[72] Maciejewski ML, Arterburn DE, Van Scoyoc L, Smith VA, Yancy WS, Weidenbacher HJ, et al. Bariatric surgery and long-term durability of weight loss. JAMA surgery. 2016 Nov 1;**151**(11):1046-1055

[73] Cooper TC, Simmons EB, Webb K, Burns JL, Kushner RF. Trends in weight regain following Roux-en-Y gastric bypass (RYGB) bariatric surgery. Obesity Surgery. 2015;**25**(8):1474-1481. Epub 2015/01/18. DOI: 10.1007/s11695-014-1560-z

[74] Freire RH, Borges MC, Alvarez-Leite JI, Toulson Davisson Correia MI. Food quality, physical activity, and nutritional follow-up as determinant of weight regain after Roux-en-Y gastric bypass. Nutrition. 2012;**28**(1):53-58. Epub 2011/09/03. DOI: 10.1016/j.nut.2011.01.011

[75] van der Burgh Y, Boerboom A, de Boer H, Witteman B, Berends F, Hazebroek E. Weight loss and malnutrition after conversion of the primary Roux-en-Y gastric bypass to distal gastric bypass in patients with morbid obesity. Surgery for Obesity and Related Diseases. 2020 Mar 1;**16**(3):381-388

[76] Sugerman HJ, Kellum JM, DeMaria EJ. Conversion of proximal to distal gastric bypass for failed gastric bypass for superobesity. Journal of Gastrointestinal Surgery. 1997 Dec;**1**(6):5171-5178

[77] Shin RD, Goldberg MB, Shafran AS, Shikora SA, Majumdar MC, Shikora SA. Revision of Roux-en-Y gastric bypass with limb distalization for inadequate weight loss or weight regain. Obesity Surgery. 2019 Mar;**29**(3):811-818

[78] Ghiassi S, Higa K, Chang S, Ma P, Lloyd A, Boone K, et al. Conversion of standard Roux-en-Y gastric bypass to distal bypass for weight loss failure and metabolic syndrome: 3-year follow-up and evolution of technique to reduce nutritional complications. Surgery for Obesity and Related Diseases. 2018 May 1;**14**(5):554-561

[79] Wang A, Poliakin L, Sundaresan N, Vijayanagar V, Abdurakhmanov A, Thompson KJ, et al. The role of total alimentary limb length in Roux-en-Y gastric bypass–a systematic review. Surgery for Obesity and Related Diseases. 2021 Aug 30

[80] Amor IB, Petrucciani N, Kassir R, Malyshev E, Mazoyer C, Korkmaz C, et al. Midterm outcomes of gastric pouch resizing for weight regain after roux-en-Y

gastric bypass. Obesity Surgery. 2020 Jul;**30**(7):2723-2728

[81] León F, Maiz C, Daroch D, Quezada N, Gabrielli M, Muñoz C, et al. Laparoscopic hand-sewn revisional gastrojejunal plication for weight loss failure after Roux-en-Y gastric bypass. Obesity Surgery. 2015 Apr;**25**(4):744-749

[82] Siilin H, Wanders A, Gustavsson S, Sundbom M. The proximal gastric pouch invariably contains acid-producing parietal cells in Roux-en-Y gastric bypass. Obesity surgery. 2005 Jun;**15**(6):771-777

[83] Dapri G, Cadière GB, Himpens J. Laparoscopic placement of non-adjustable silicone ring for weight regain after Roux-en-Y gastric bypass. Obesity surgery. 2009 May;**19**(5):650-654

[84] Bessler M, Daud A, DiGiorgi MF, Inabnet WB, Schrope B, Olivero-Rivera L, et al. Adjustable gastric banding as revisional bariatric procedure after failed gastric bypass—intermediate results. Surgery for Obesity and Related Diseases. 2010 Jan 1;**6**(1):31-35

[85] Jirapinyo P, Slattery J, Ryan MB, Dayyeh BA, Lautz DB, Thompson CC. Evaluation of an endoscopic suturing device for transoral outlet reduction in patients with weight regain following Roux-en-Y gastric bypass. Endoscopy. 2013 Jul;**45**(07):532-536

[86] Gallo AS, DuCoin CG, Berducci MA, Nino DF, Almadani M, Sandler BJ, Horgan S, Jacobsen GR. Endoscopic revision of gastric bypass: Holy Grail or Epic fail?. Surgical endoscopy. 2016 Sep;**30**(9):3922-3927

[87] Kim HJ, Madan A, Fenton-Lee D. Does patient compliance with follow-up influence weight loss after gastric bypass surgery? A systematic review and meta-analysis. Obesity surgery. 2014 Apr;**24**(4):647-651

[88] Conceição E, Pinto-Bastos A, de Lourdes M, Brandão I, Teixeira C, Machado PPP. Psychological, behavioral, and weight-related aspects of patients undergoing reoperative bariatric surgery after gastric band: Comparison with primary surgery patients. Surgery for Obesity and Related Diseases. 2018;**14**(5):603-610. DOI: 10.1016/j.soard.2018.02.011

Chapter 3

Laparoscopic Sleeve Gastrectomy – Technical Tips and Pitfalls

Muhammed Said Dalkılıç, Mehmet Gençtürk, Merih Yılmaz, Abdullah Şişik, Hasan Erdem, Selim Sözen and Burhan Hakan Kanat

Abstract

Today, bariatric surgery is the most effective treatment for obesity, and the techniques continue to evolve. Laparoscopic sleeve gastrectomy, which is only one step of biliopancreatic diversion/duodenal switch surgery, has become the most common bariatric procedure due to its efficacy when performed alone. Additionally, the rate of complications has decreased as a result of increased technical experience and the development of stapler technology. The widespread adoption of laparoscopic sleeve gastrectomy is also attributable to its technical simplicity. Although it is assumed to be a simple procedure, mistakes at specific stages significantly increase the risk of complications. We focus on our method in detail, including all operative steps, which we believe is the simplest and most effective technique after performing over 5000 surgeries at our institution. Paying attention to the sleeve size, selecting the appropriate stapler, not narrowing the incisura angularis, resecting the fundus without getting too close to the esophagus, creating a smooth, non-rotating staple line, and suturing the staple line are highlighted.

Keywords: obesity, bariatric surgery, gastrectomy, stomach stapling

1. Introduction

Gastrectomy for weight loss was first described by Marceau et al. in 1993 as a restrictive component of biliopancreatic diversion [1]. Then they described the vertical sleeve gastrectomy as the first step of the biliopancreatic diversion-duodenal switch procedure in 1998 [2].

Unfortunately, the laparoscopic duodenal switch was associated with significant complications, especially in patients with high body mass index [3]. Thus, Gagner et al. performed laparoscopic sleeve gastrectomy (LSG) as the initial stage of a two-staged approach before BPD/DS and Roux-en-Y gastric bypass to optimize the performance status of patients at high surgical risk or extremely obese [4, 5]. Many of these patients achieved adequate weight loss and improvement in medical comorbidities

 IntechOpen

after the first sleeve gastrectomy, and the second stage was rarely required. Therefore, LSG has evolved into a stand-alone weight loss procedure over time.

Long-term data show that LSG is as similar in weight loss and comorbidity resolution as the Roux-en-Y gastric bypass and has similar mortality and morbidity rates [6]. It is now the most commonly performed bariatric procedure worldwide, owing to its technical simplicity, short learning curve, and effectiveness [7].

The procedure has not been standardized yet. Different technical nuances can be seen at various points throughout the process. In this section, we focus on our method in detail, including all operative steps, which we believe is the simplest and most effective technique after performing over 5000 surgeries at our institution.

2. Mechanism of action

The efficacy of the laparoscopic sleeve gastrectomy leading to sustained weight loss and improvement in comorbidities results from various mechanisms. First, owing to the reduction in stomach volume, there is a dramatic decrease in alimentary intake. Second, the orexigenic hormone ghrelin, which stimulates food intake, fat deposition, and the release of growth hormone, has dropped significantly. One of the primary goals of LSG is to eliminate the fundus, which is the primary source of ghrelin. Moreover, Glucagon-like-peptide-1, Peptide YY, and pancreatic polypeptide may also be factors involved in the mechanism of weight loss [8, 9]. Apparently, this mechanism is most likely multifactorial and still not fully clarified.

2.1 Preoperative considerations

LSG surgery is recommended for patients with a BMI greater than 40 kg/m^2 or a BMI greater than 35 kg/m^2 and co-morbid diseases such as type II diabetes, hypertension, obstructive sleep apnea (OSA), non-alcoholic fatty liver disease, osteoarthritis, hyperlipidemia, or heart disease.

All patients considering bariatric surgery should undergo an adequate preoperative evaluation and workup including lab tests (complete blood count, basic metabolic panel, coagulation panel, HgA1C, thyroid function tests, vitamins, B-HCG for women), chest X-ray, and ECG [10].

Although upper GI endoscopy and abdominal ultrasonography are not routinely recommended, they contain important information that may affect the surgical plan. Concomitant hiatal hernia, esophagitis, H. pylori, and occult malignancies can all be evaluated using esophagogastroduodenoscopy. On the other hand, ultrasonography provides information about cholelithiasis, steatohepatitis, and other abdominal pathologies.

The evaluation of patients with gastroesophageal reflux preoperatively is controversial due to the conflicting results of LSG on reflux symptoms. There are studies in the literature claiming that LSG either improves or worsens reflux [11, 12]. Due to the risk of worsening the current situation and the need for revisional surgery, LSG is not the best option for patients with significant gastroesophageal reflux disease (GERD). The ASMBS released a statement declaring that severe GERD symptoms and Barrett's esophagus are relative contraindications to LSG [13]. Roux en Y gastric bypass, which has long been used as an anti-reflux procedure, should be recommended for this population.

Increased reflux symptoms after LSG can be associated with a concomitant hiatal hernia. There is an emerging consensus on concomitant hiatal repair [14]. According to the International Consensus Conference on Sleeve Gastrectomy, 84% of bariatric surgeons believe it should be repaired if present [15].

Smoking cessation and OSA management are critical for preventing respiratory complications in bariatric patients whose oxygen delivery to tissues may be compromised.

Furthermore, the following elements must be addressed: evaluation and optimization of comorbidities; consultation with a dietician, psychiatrist, and endocrinologist; and informed consent and thorough education regarding expectations [7].

2.2 Anesthesia

The procedure requires general endotracheal tube anesthesia. The anesthesiologist should be prepared for the possibility of difficult intubation, which is common in obese patients, and should have a flexible bronchoscope to assist with endotracheal tube placement.

3. Patient positioning and operative field

The patient is positioned in reverse Trendelenburg and supine with both arms abducted and the legs split (French position). The patient is fixed to the operation table from both legs and the infraumblical site. The surgical covers and instruments are placed after the iodine wash of the abdominal skin. A 5-mm vessel sealer is prepared for dissection. A urinary catheter is not routinely placed. Patients are administered antithrombotic medication (enoxaparin) 12 hours before surgery in addition to sequential pneumatic compression stockings and prophylactic antibiotics.

The surgeon starts on the patient's right during trocar placement and then stands between the legs at the center. The assistant holds the camera with the left hand and uses grasper with the right hand on the patient's left and a nurse on the patient's right (**Figure 1**).

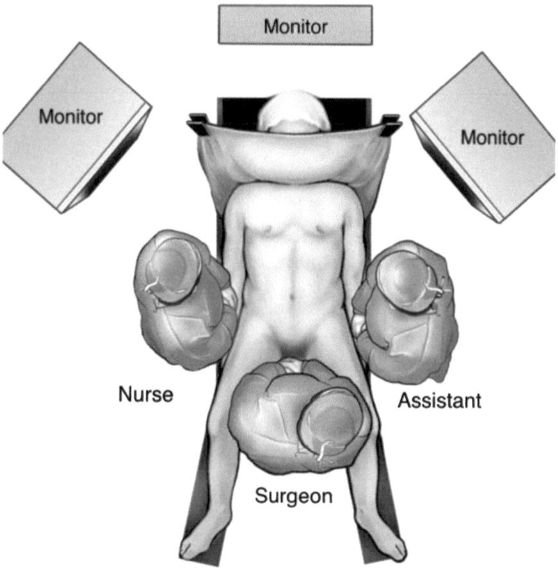

Figure 1.
Operative positioning.

3.1 Surgical technique

3.1.1 Trocar placement and Pneumoperitoneum

Pneumoperitoneum can be established with a variety of techniques (open, visualizing trocars or Veress needle), but we prefer the direct entry method. Although the direct entry method has a long learning curve and requires experience, it is a fast and safe method when performed by experienced surgeons. Only five patients in our series had lacerations in the gastric serosa, and one patient with extensive intra-abdominal adhesions had full-thickness colon injury, which was noticed and repaired during the surgery (**Figure 2**).

The first trocar for a 10-mm camera is placed 10–12 cm below the xiphoid, and CO_2 is insufflated up to 14–16 mm Hg. A laparoscope with 30° camera is introduced, and the abdominal cavity is inspected to rule out injury from the trocar and any other anatomic abnormalities such as adhesions. Three more trocars and a retractor are placed as shown in **Figure 3**:

1. A 15-mm trocar in the right upper quadrant provides passage of the black staple load. The remainder of the cartridges (purple) fit through a 12-mm port. This is also used for the left-hand working port.

2. A 5-mm trocar in the left upper quadrant on the midclavicular line. This working port is for the surgeon's right hand.

3. A 5-mm trocar in the lateral left upper quadrant on the anterior axillary line. It is used by the first assistant for retraction.

4. The Nathanson® liver retractor is placed via an additional 5-mm incision in the superior epigastrium.

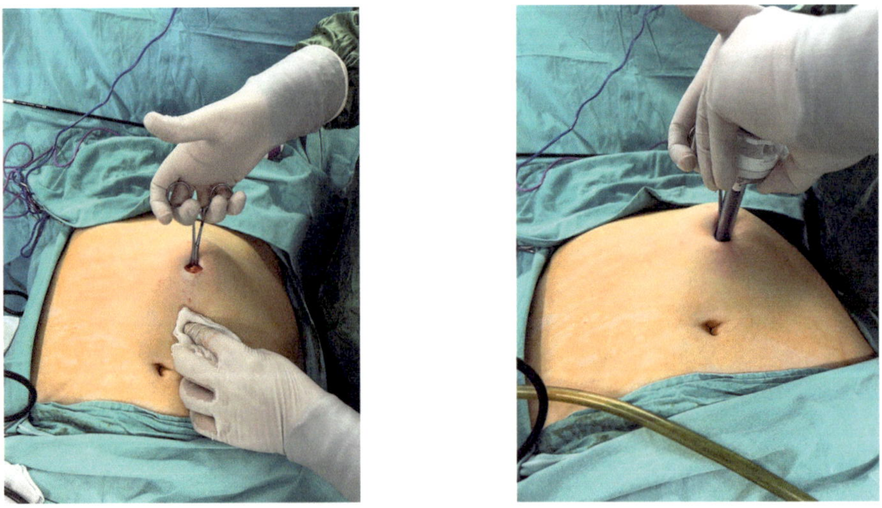

Figure 2.
Direct entry of the camera trocar (left-handed surgeon). The surgeon grasps the fascia with a towel clamp and lifts it upward to avoid any intraabdominal injury.

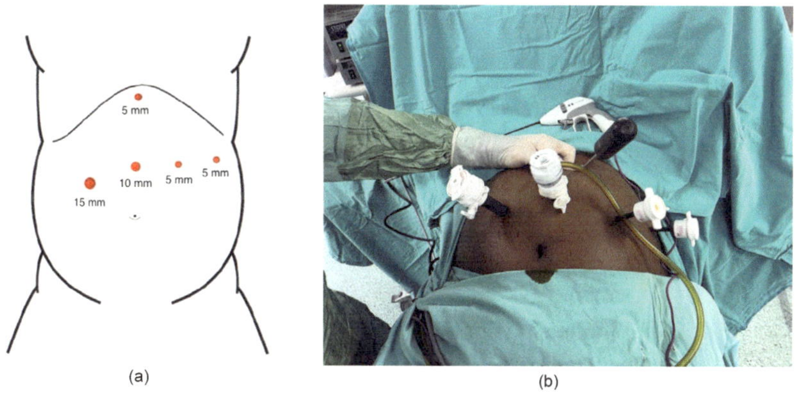

Figure 3.
(a, b) Trocar placement.

With the surgeon's command, the orogastric tube is placed to evacuate the stomach and should be taken to 30–35 cm of the esophagus.

Tip: The entry point of the camera trocar should not be adjusted to the umbilicus, but to the xiphoid, which is a more reliable and stable mark. The location of the umbilicus may vary depending on the patient's BMI and anatomical features. Also, the location of the umbilicus has changed in patients who have undergone abdominoplasty. If the camera trocar is inserted lower than it should be, fundus dissection will be difficult, especially in patients with high BMI.

Tip: Adequate aspiration of the stomach provides serious convenience, especially during fundus and left crus dissection. Dissection can be difficult while the tube is in the stomach.

Pitfall: To avoid any injury, a nasogastric or orogastric tube should not be inserted without the knowledge of the surgeon. In case of carelessness or miscommunication, the tube is fired between the staplers.

3.1.2 Gastrocolic omentum dissection

Dissection begins from the corpus-antrum junction of the greater curvature. The gastrocolic omentum is divided off the greater curvature of the stomach with the energy device on the surgeon's right hand, beginning approximately 3–4 cm proximal to the pylorus and proceeding to the angle of His, completely mobilizing the greater curve (**Figure 4**).

Tip: The surgeon's left hand pulls the stomach to the upside while the assistant catches the gastrocolic ligament and pulls gently to the downside. It allows working close to the great curvature, which reduces the risk of bleeding from gastroepiploic vessels and facilitates specimen extraction at the end of the operation (**Figure 5**).

Pitfall: If a dissection close to the stomach is not performed, bleeding from the gastroepiploic vessels may occur and take time to stop .

3.1.3 Posterior adhesions dissection

All posterior attachments to the pancreas must be divided, taking care not to injure the lesser curvature and left gastric vessels because the blood supply to the sleeve originates solely from the lesser curvature vasculature.

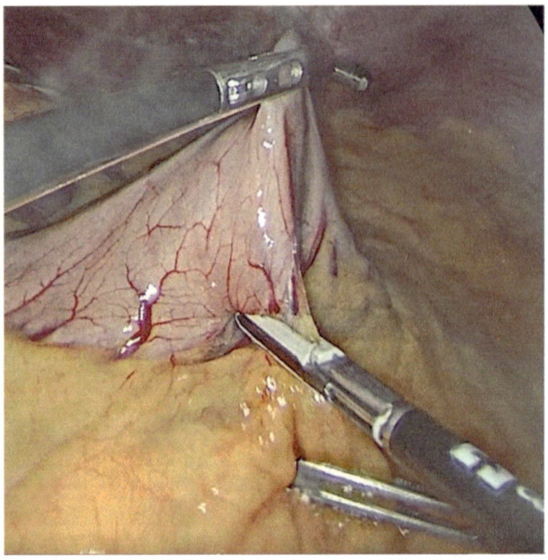

(a)

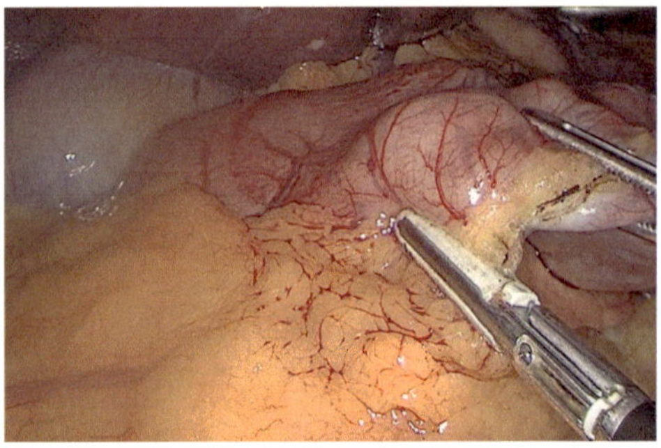

(b)

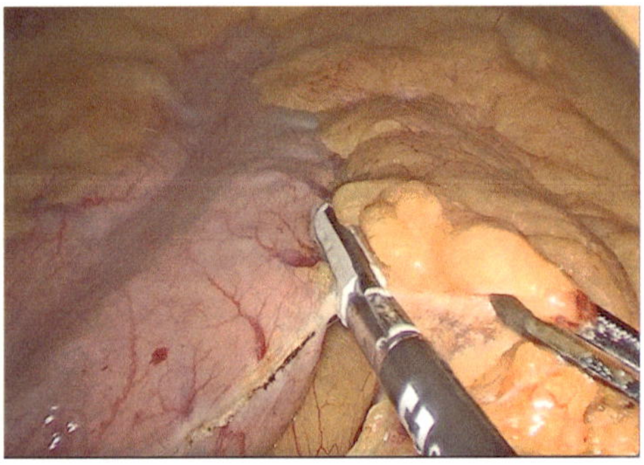

(C)

Figure 4.
(a-c) Gastrocolic Omentum Dissection (a) shows the first movement to enter the lesser sac via stomach traction and omentum contra-traction. Surgeon separates the omentum up to 3 cm proximal to the pylorus in (b). Dissection is continued close to the stomach, along the greater curvature to the angle of His in (c).

Tip: The most efficient maneuver to achieve adequate exposure for the posterior dissection is to retract the posterior aspect of the stomach upward with two graspers.

Pitfall: It is important to divide these attachments before stapling because these attachments can tear and create bleeding. However, left gastric and splenic vessels should be preserved (**Figure 6**).

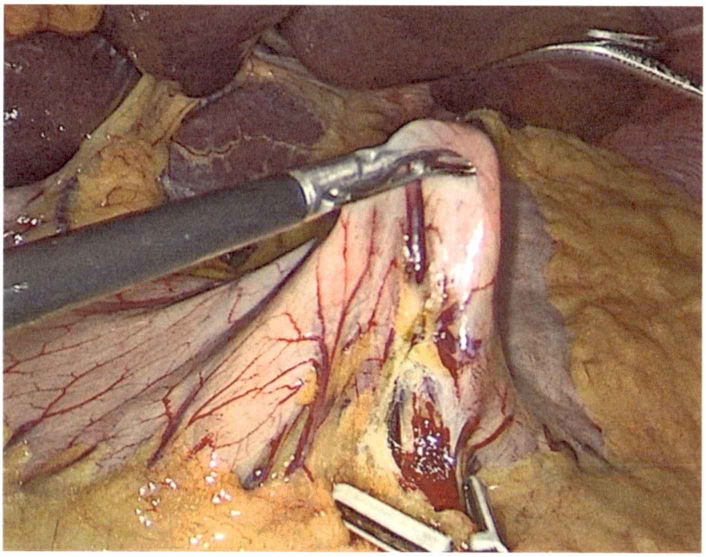

Figure 5.
Bleeding from the gastrocolic omentum.

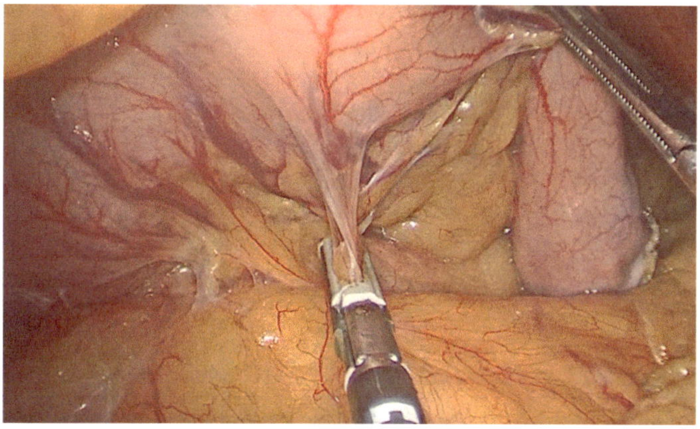

Figure 6.
Posterior Dissection (Retracting the stomach upwards with two graspers provides an adequate exposure).

3.1.4 Fundus dissection

The entire fundus should be freed posteriorly from the left crus. In order to properly diagnose a hiatal hernia and ensure that no fundus tissue is left behind, the left crus and gastroesophageal junction must be fully exposed. A gastric fat pad (especially if it is large and complicates the resection) can be resected.

Tip: The surgeon pulls the stomach slightly to the right-downward via the left hand, and the first assistant gently performs various maneuvers, such as pulling the fundus up or to the right to provide the best visualization. This is the most efficient maneuver to achieve adequate exposure for the fundus dissection.

Pitfall: During this portion of the procedure, care should be taken to avoid excessive traction and bleeding from short gastric and splenic vessels. Possible bleeding in

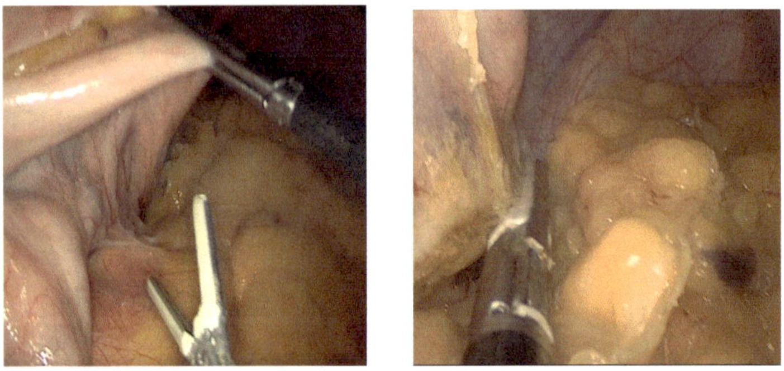

(a) (b)

Figure 7.
(a, b) Traction of the fundus (The surgeon pulls the stomach slightly to the right-downward, and the assistant does the active maneuvers).

this splenic region can be difficult to control, especially in patients with a higher BMI. A sponge can be placed in this area to control the bleeding (**Figure 7**).

3.1.5 Orogastric tube insertion

Although the preferred orogastric tube size varies between 32 Fr and 42 Fr, the average bougie size used by experts today is 36–37 French [6].

Before the first staple firing, a 36 French orogastric tube is placed by the anesthesia team. The surgeon can guide the bougie using graspers for proper placement. The tube is positioned in the antrum along the lesser curvature and not passed through the pylorus.

Tip: The stomach should be placed in its anatomical position, and the orogastric tube should stay parallel to lesser curvature. Also, stretching the stomach by excessive pushing of the tube compromises the straightness of the stapler line (**Figure 8**).

3.1.6 Transection

Transection of the stomach begins on the antrum 3–4 cm proximal to the pylorus with a black 60-mm-long cartridge with an articulating stapler. Transection of the

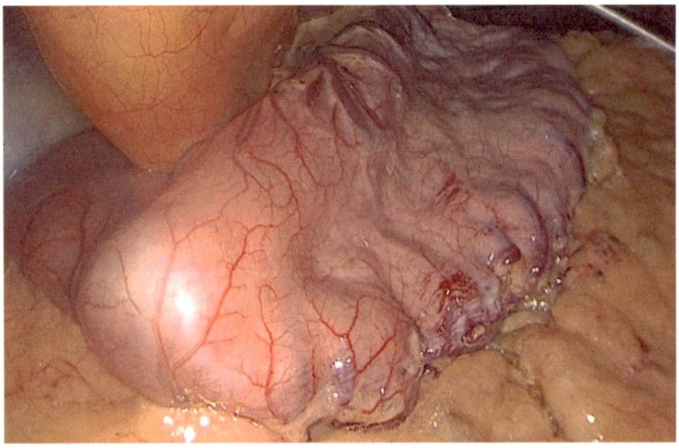

Figure 8.
Orogastric tube insertion (No excessive stretching of the stomach).

stomach should begin no less than 3 cm proximal to the pylorus [7]. Then purple 60-mm-long cartridges are used for the remainder. The thickness of the stomach tissue becomes thinner from the antrum to the fundus. Therefore, surgeons choose the tallest cartridges (black, green) at the antrum level, and while going proximal in the stomach, shorter (purple, blue, and golden) cartridges are chosen. It is crucial to ensure adequate resection of the fundus. Approximately 75–80% of the stomach is resected.

Tip: The incisura angularis should not be narrowed during stapler placement, the stomach should be laid in its anatomical position with equal apposition of the anterior and posterior aspects of the sleeve, and the orogastric tube should not be approached with excessive traction. This technique creates a straight staple line resistant to strictures, kinks, twists, and leaks.

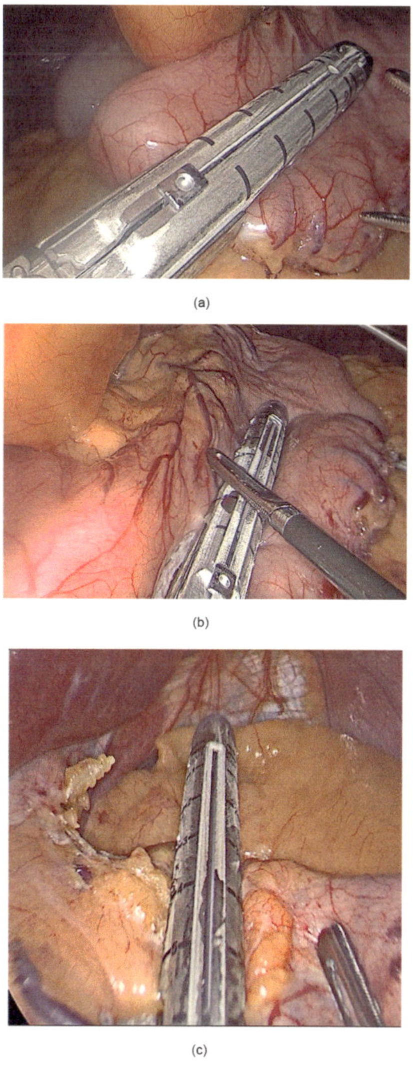

Figure 9.
a-c Staplings (Surgeon avoids narrowing the incisura angularis during the first stapling as shown in (a) and makes control with a clamp to be sure during the second stapling in (b). Last staple that is not adjacent to the esophagus is shown in (c)).

Tip: Gastric tissue thickens due to contractions in some cases, making transection difficult. In our experience, administering intravenous Hyoscine butylbromide (Scopolamine) before transection, which reduces contractions with its anticholinergic effect, may result in a straighter and smoother staple line in these patients. However, there are no clinical studies to back up this assertion (**Figure 9**).

Pitfall: The last fire has to be done 0.5–1 cm lateral to the His angle to avoid the risk of ischemia-related leak and fistulas (**Figure 10**).

3.1.7 Bleeding control and staple line reinforcement

Staple line bleeding (SLB) is a common intraoperative complication following resection in LSG [16]. A hemostatic clip (10 mm) is a quick and simple tool for controlling bleeding, particularly oozing. Clips are also used at stapler transition points as they are considered potentially vulnerable areas, though this has not been proven.

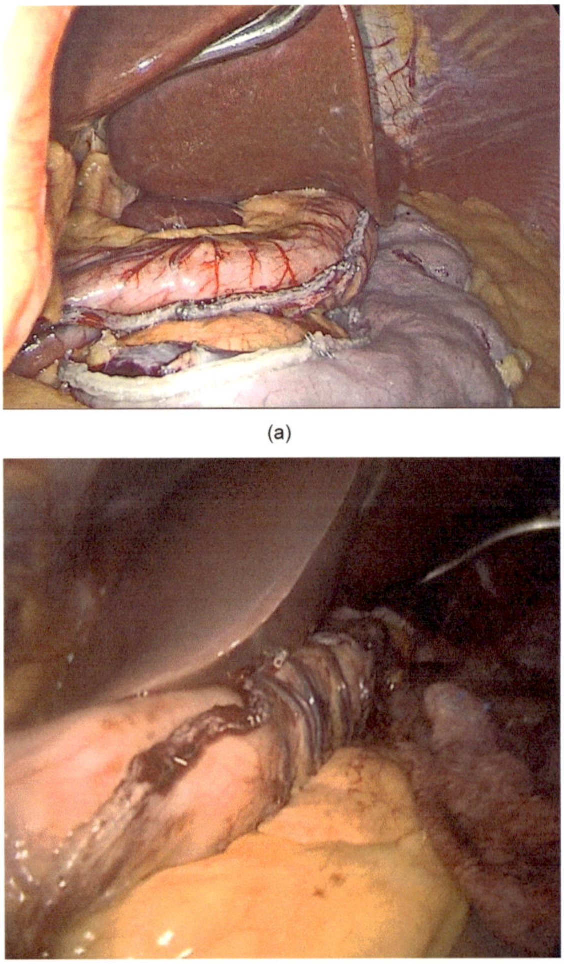

(a)

(b)

Figure 10.
(a, b) (a) shows a straight and smooth staple line that should be aimed. The false stapling technique results in an irregular staple line that is prone to complications (b).

Staple line reinforcement is a controversial step of the procedure. Although it has not been demonstrated that routine reinforcement of the staple line is necessary, we usually reinforce the staple line with sutures in our practice. During this process, we prefer to sew the dissected omentum majus line to the stapler line. With this reinforcement, we hope to reduce complications including leakage and stenosis (due to the formation of a twist or kink) and most notably, bleeding. The decision to reinforce should be based on the stapler used and the patient's condition. According to recent studies on bariatric surgery, the following risk factors for postoperative bleeding are stated: male sex, >45 years of age, body mass index <40 kg/m^2, cardiovascular disease, and current procedure of LSG, bougie size, prior cardiac procedure, hypertension, renal insufficiency, therapeutic anticoagulation, diabetes, obstructive sleep apnea, and operative length [17, 18].

Perioperative control of blood pressure is another important measure to prevent bleeding. Because it is assumed that some of the bleeding is due to the sudden increase in blood pressure during the operation or in the post-anesthesia care unit [19] (**Figure 11**). It should be ensured that the blood pressure is kept below a certain level, especially from the firing stage to the early postoperative period. Karaman et al. found that keeping the systolic blood pressure below 120 mm Hg during surgery reduced staple line bleeding [9]. In our practice, we keep our systolic blood pressure target around 100–110 mm Hg throughout the surgery. Blood pressure control is achieved by titration of remifentanil infusion and, if necessary, glyceryl trinitrate infusion is started (**Figure 12**).

3.1.8 Drain placement

We routinely place a soft drain to take early measures for bleeding, but it is known that many surgeons have recently abandoned the use of drains (**Figure 13**).

3.1.9 Resected stomach (specimen) extraction

The specimen is extracted with jaws grasper through the-15 mm trocar incision under direct visualization.

Pitfall: Specimen removal can be quite difficult, especially in large stomachs, and will result in a rupture if the correct gentle maneuvers are not performed with patience.

Tip: To prevent this situation, the specimen should be removed by pulling the greater curvature, not the staple line, because the staple line is weaker (**Figure 14**).

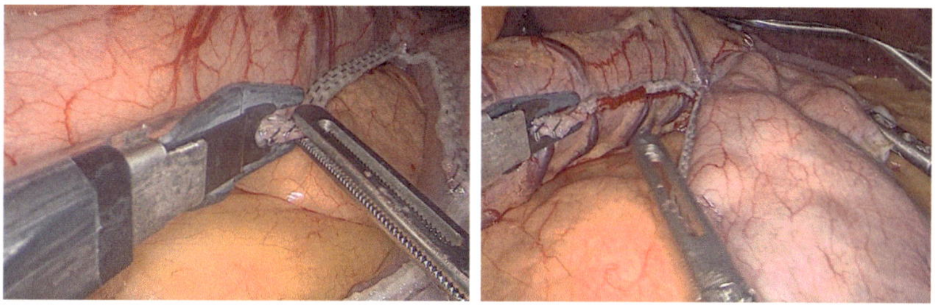

(a) (b)

Figure 11.
a,b Clips to the staple line. A hemostatic clip is a straightforward tool for bleeding and also can be used at staple transition points for reinforcement.

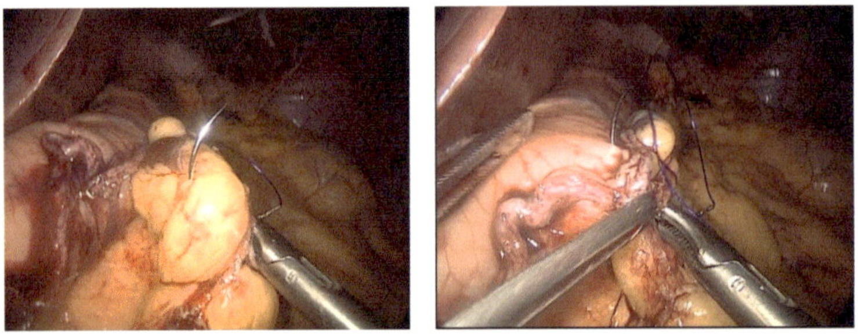

Figure 12.
Omentopexy and sewing.

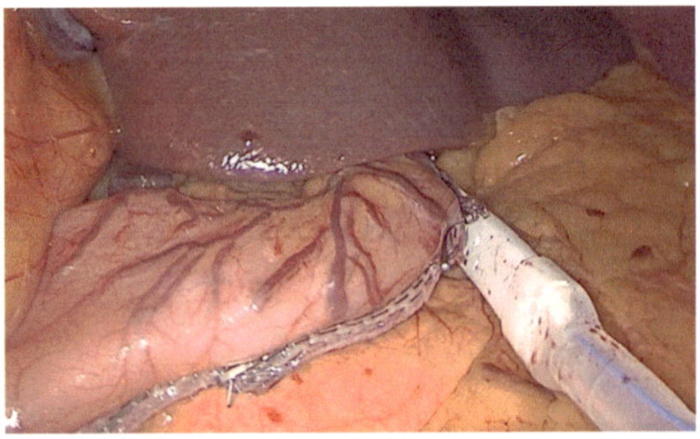

Figure 13.
Drain.

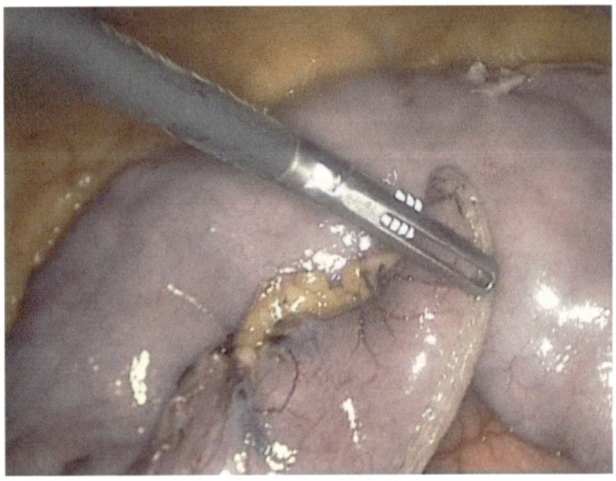

Figure 14.
Specimen removal with a jaws grasper.

3.1.10 Closure of Trocar sites

The 15- and 10-mm trocar fascial defects are closed with a suture passer.

Pitfall: If not repaired, trocar site hernias may occur, mainly due to 15-mm fascial defects (**Figure 15**).

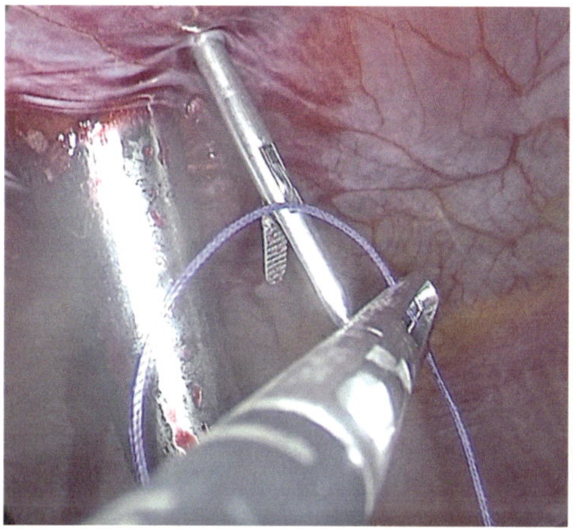

Figure 15.
Fascial closure with a suture passer device.

3.2 Early postoperative care

It is critical to resume analgesics and antiemetics in the recovery unit. To prevent vomiting or retching, aggressive nausea prevention and early mobilization are provided. The combination of antiemetics such as ondansetron and metoclopramide with multimodal analgesia is effective.

In our practice, patients are mobilized 2–4 hours after surgery. After the anesthetic drugs have worn off, small sips of water are taken. Clear liquids are usually started on the first postoperative day, followed by a high-protein liquid diet on the second day. The majority of patients are ready for discharge home on the second day. Daily micronutrient supplements are required due to inadequate dietary intake. Anticoagulation prophylaxis is provided for 2 weeks after discharge. A proton pump inhibitor is recommended for 3 months.

Many obese patients have OSA, and if their personal device is present, it is safe and preferred. However, some may require continuous pulse oximetry and positive airway pressure in the ICU following surgery.

CRP levels and complete blood count are highly correlated with postoperative complications and can be taken every 24 hours.

The postoperative diet is varied. Usually, practices begin with clear liquids, increasing the volume gradually. Intake should be in small portions. The daily intake goal is 2 L. If the patient tolerates this, liquid foods such as milk and yogurt can be safely started without delay. After 1–2 weeks, patients progress to a mashed or pure diet. It is recommended to separate liquids from solids. After 2 weeks, patients can start a soft diet. The solid foods are started at 1 month [7].

4. Summary

Although LSG can be performed with different technical methods at various stages, to avoid postoperative complications and obtain the best weight loss results, it is necessary to pay attention to the following key points:

1. Pay attention to the sleeve size, which determines the weight loss results.
2. Choose the stapler suitable for tissue thickness.
3. Avoid narrowing the incisura angularis.
4. Resect the fundus as much as possible without getting too close to the esophagus.
5. Create a smooth non-rotating staple line.
6. Reinforce the staple line.

Author details

Muhammed Said Dalkılıç[1], Mehmet Gençtürk[2], Merih Yılmaz[2], Abdullah Şişik[2], Hasan Erdem[2], Selim Sözen[3] and Burhan Hakan Kanat[4]*

1 Marmara University, School of Medicine, Department of General Surgery, Istanbul, Turkey

2 Obesity Clinic, Istanbul, Turkey

3 Sozen Surgery Clinic, Tekirdağ, Turkey

4 Malatya Turugt Özal University, School of Medicine, Department of General Surgery, Malatya, Turkey

*Address all correspondence to: burhankanat@hotmail.com

References

[1] Marceau P, Biron S, St. Georges R, Duclos M, Potvin M, Bourque R-A. Biliopancreatic diversion with gastrectomy as surgical treatment of morbid obesity. Obesity Surgery. 1993;**3**:29-35

[2] Marceau P, Hould FS, Simard S, et al. Biliopancreatic diversion with duodenal switch. World Journal of Surgery. 1998;**22**:947-954

[3] Gumbs AA, Gagner M, Dankin G, et al. Sleeve gastrectomy for morbid obesity. Obesity Surgery. 2007;**17**(7):962-969

[4] Ren CJ, Patterson E, Gagner M. Early results of laparoscopic biliopancreatic diversion with duodenal switch: A case series of 40 consecutive patients. Obesity Surgery. 2000;**10**(6):514-523; discussion 524. DOI: 10.1381/096089200321593715

[5] Regan JP, Inabnet WB, Gagner M, Pomp A. Early experience with two-stage laparoscopic Roux-en-Y gastric bypass as an alternative in the super-super obese patient. Obesity Surgery. 2003;**13**(6):861-864. DOI: 10.1381/096089203322618669

[6] Shoar S, Saber AS. Long-term and midterm outcomes of laparoscopic sleeve gastrectomy versus Roux-en-Y gastric bypass: A systematic review and meta-analysis of comparative studies. Surgery for Obesity and Related Diseases. 2017;**13**:170-180

[7] Chung AY, Thompson R, Overby DW, Duke MC, Farrell TM. Sleeve gastrectomy: Surgical tips. Journal of Laparoendoscopic & Advanced Surgical Techniques. Part A. 2018;**28**(8):930-937. DOI: 10.1089/lap.2018.0392 Epub 2018 Jul 13

[8] Climaco K, Ahnfeldt E. Laparoscopic vertical sleeve gastrectomy. Surgical Clinics of North America. 2021;**101**(2):177-188. DOI: 10.1016/j.suc.2020.12.015

[9] Telem DA, Gould J, Pesta C, et al. American society for metabolic and bariatric surgery: A care pathway development for laparoscopic sleeve gastrectomy. Surgery for Obesity and Related Diseases. 2017;**13**(5):742-749

[10] Rebecchi F, Allaix ME, Giaccone C, et al. Gastroesophageal reflux disease and laparoscopic sleeve gastrectomy: A physiopathologic evaluation. Annals of Surgery. 2014;**260**:909-915

[11] Stenard F, Iannelli A. Laparoscopic sleeve gastrectomy and gastroesophageal reflux. World Journal of Gastroenterology. 2015;**21**:10348-10357

[12] Ali M, El Chaar M, Ghiassi S, et al. American society for metabolic and bariatric surgery updated position statement on sleeve gastrectomy as a bariatric procedure. Surgery for Obesity and Related Diseases. 2017;**13**(10):1652-1657

[13] Clapp B, Liggett E, Barrientes A, Aguirre K, Marwaha V, Tyroch A. Concomitant hiatal hernia repair with sleeve gastrectomy: A 5-year analysis. Journal of the Society of Laparoendoscopic Surgeons. 2020;**24**(4):e2020.00066. DOI: 10.4293/JSLS.2020.00066

[14] Gagner M, Hutchinson C, Rosenthal R. Fifth International Consensus Conference: Current status of sleeve gastrectomy. Surgery for Obesity and Related Diseases. 2016;**12**(4):750-756

[15] Chakravartty S, Sarma DR, Chang A, Patel AG. Staple line bleeding

in sleeve gastrectomy-a simple and cost-effective solution. Obesity Surgery. 2016;**26**(7):1422-1428. DOI: 10.1007/s11695-015-1986-y

[16] Straatman J, Verhaak T, Demirkiran A, Harlaar NJ, Cense HA, Jonker FHW. Dutch audit for treatment of obesity (DATO) research group. Risk factors for postoperative bleeding in bariatric surgery. Surgery for Obesity and Related Diseases. 2022;**18**(8):1057-1065. DOI: 10.1016/j.soard.2022.05.010 Epub 2022 May 18

[17] Mocanu V, Dang J, Ladak F, Switzer N, Birch DW, Karmali S. Predictors and outcomes of bleed after sleeve gastrectomy: An analysis of the MBSAQIP data registry. Surgery for Obesity and Related Diseases. 2019;**15**(10):1675-1681. DOI: 10.1016/j.soard.2019.07.017 Epub 2019 Aug 10

[18] Janik MR, Rogula T, Kowalewski P, Walędziak M, Matłok M, Brągoszewski J, et al. Case-control study of postoperative blood pressure in patients with hemorrhagic complications after laparoscopic sleeve gastrectomy and matched controls. Obesity Surgery. 2017;**27**(7):1849-1853. DOI: 10.1007/s11695-017-2569-x

[19] Karaman K, Aziret M, Ercan M, Ebiloglu T, Karadeniz U, Bostanci EB. A preventive strategy for staple line bleeding in morbidly obese patients undergoing sleeve gastrectomy. Journal of Laparoendoscopic & Advanced Surgical Techniques. Part A. 2017;**27**(10):1015-1021. DOI: 10.1089/lap.2017.0386 Epub 2017 Aug 22

Section 2

Post Bariatric Surgery

Chapter 4

Predicting Factors for Weight Regain after Bariatric Surgery

Ivaylo Tzvetkov

Abstract

Weight regain (WR) after bariatric surgery (BS) is emerging as a common clinical problem due to the increase in the number of procedures performed worldwide. Weight regain is defined as regain of weight that occurs few years after the bariatric procedure and successful achievement of the initial weight loss. Causes of WR following BS are multifactorial and can be categorized into two main groups: patient and surgical-specific causes. Several mechanisms contribute to WR following BS. These include hormonal mechanisms, nutritional non-adherence, physical inactivity, mental health causes, maladaptive eating, surgical techniques, and the selection criteria for the weight loss procedure. Higher preoperative BMI seems to be associated with WR and worse weight loss results in a long term. Patients with baseline BMI ≥ 50 kg/m^2 are more likely to have significant WR, while those with BMI < 50 are likely to continue losing weight at 12 months post-surgery. The aim of the chapter is to discuss and reveal all main factors, which may contribute to weight regain after bariatric surgery and emphasize how multifactorial assessment and long-term support/follow-up of patients by key medical professionals can diminish the side effects of weight regain.

Keywords: bariatric surgery, weight loss, weight regain, excessive weight loss, eating disorders, gastric bypass, sleeve gastrectomy, one anastomosis gastric bypass

1. Introduction

There are several definitions of Obesity worldwide [1]. Interestingly, it is considered as a kind of malnutrition nowadays. Morbid Obesity is mostly a problem in high-income countries, according to statistical data with prevalence of countries in North America. However, overweight and obesity are a socially significant growing problem in low- and middle-income countries also. The estimated increase of Obesity among children is more than 30% higher in those countries than in developed countries in the last 10 years. The data confirm that 1.9 billion adults worldwide were overweight in 2016, with 650 million being Obese. People who are obese have much higher risks of many serious health problems than nonobese people [2, 3]. Obesity affects every system of the body. The results of outcome of bariatric surgery (BS) confirm the positive effects of surgery over such conditions as Diabetes type 2 (DT2), fatty liver disease, cancer. There is evidence for improvement of thyroid function, heart function, fertility, and sexual function in patients who have had weight loss surgery. More than

50 bariatric procedures have been proposed and implemented so far. As a result of time and trial, several procedures have been established as standards. The final goal of those procedures is for the Morbid Obese patient to achieve at least a loss of 50–70% of excess weight [EWL] or about 20–30% loss of his initial weight. Some authors consider a successful outcome, when achieving a Body Mass Index [BMI] < 35 kg/m^2 2 years after surgery in those patients. However, the BMI as a criterion for a successful outcome after B/M surgery is under debate due to several reports that even patients with BMI of 32.0 can benefit from Metabolic surgery. So, we think that the quality benchmark for outcome of any M/B surgical procedure should be a combination of percentage of EWL in short and mid-term, extrapolated with percentage of WR in a long term—about 10 years after surgery. We support the suggestion of SOS study [4, 5] that patients should not regain more than 20–25% of their lost weight within 10 years after the primary procedure. Several studies confirm average weight regain of 12% of total body weight in patients who underwent Roux en Y Gastric bypass (RYGB), while those reported for Sleeve Gastrectomy (SG) were variable, ranging from 6% at as early as 2 years post-surgery to 76% at 6 years post-surgery [6–8]. Morbid Obesity, like other chronic diseases, persists for prolonged durations and requires a continuous close follow-up to reassess the efficacy of treatments, including Bariatric/Metabolic surgery. Most of the reports for very good and excellent results after weight loss surgery [WLS] are short or mid-long term up to 5 years' studies. Unfortunately, the studies, reporting results for more than 5 years after surgery, revealed a significant rate of WR in patients with Body Mass Index over 50 or history of comorbidity of more than 5 years [6, 9].

2. Definition of weight regain

The general metrics to assess the success of the surgeries includes calculating % of excessive weight loss (EWL) (>50%), % of total weight loss (TWL), and % of weight regain (WR) post-surgery. Different studies have shown a large amount of variability within these values, which have been attributed to the type of surgery, the preoperative BMI, and to the race and ethnicity that the patients belong to [2–4, 10]. Literature review studies have revealed that only a limited number of them have looked at differences in weight loss patterns across different populations and specifically in the European population, where Bariatric/Metabolic procedures are performed routinely in nowadays. However, the sustained health improvements following bariatric surgery are dependent on the individual's adherence to long-term changes in lifestyle habits [11, 12]. As a result, despite its effectiveness, weight regain after bariatric surgery is a persistent problematic issue!

The first group of patients are those who do not lose the expected or anticipated average percentage of weight following surgery, while the second group are patients who lose a successful amount of weight after Bariatric/Metabolic Surgery (B/MS), but they regain some or most of the weight 5 or more years after the initial procedure [10].

According to several authors and publications about weight loss surgery, we must make a distinction between two types of WL failure post (B/MS). The first is known as insufficient WL (IWL). The second is known as weight regain (WR). IWL is defined as excess weight loss (EWL%) of <50% at 18 months after BS. Weight regain is defined as regain of weight that occurs few years after the Bariatric procedure and successful achievement of the initial weight loss. Literature review found several definitions for WR [13–15] as:

- regaining weight reaching a body mass index (BMI) >35 after successful WL;
- an increase in BMI of ≥ 5 kg/m^2 above the nadir weight; >
- 25% EWL% regain from nadir; increase in weight of >10 kg from nadir;
- any WR or any WR after Diabetes Mellitus type 2 (DT2) remission;
- an increase of >15% of total body weight from nadir.

All those definitions describe one and the same problem: WR several years after B/MS. A robust review of the main causes, leading to that problem, is mandatory in order to answer to significant health and social issues about application of B/MS worldwide.

3. Factors for weight regain after bariatric surgery

It is difficult to outline current factors, leading to WR after B/MS. The role of those factors and their influence on patient's behavior, eating habits, and ability to keep his weight under control after the primary procedure are not well understood or investigated robustly. However, most of the published reviews confirm that they have been attributed to several surgical, biological, and behavioral factors [2, 16]. We can identify two groups of factors nowadays. The first group is of so-called non- modifiable factors as hormonal, metabolic, surgery-related [14, 17]. The second group is of so-called "modifiable behaviors," where patients should receive more support and care within 5 years after surgery by healthcare professionals. WR remains a major challenge in relation to the long-term success of B/MS [7, 8]. Although weight regain is a consistent finding among studies, there are considerable variations in the magnitude and rate of weight regain depending on factors ranging from behavioral, dietary, lifestyle, psychological, ethnic, and racial differences. Interestingly, there are studies that report an average of 56% WR weight within 10 years after primary surgery [10, 18]. A poor prognostic indicator for WR after B/MS is the slow weight loss in the first two postoperative years. Medical based evidence confirms that patients, who achieve 20–30% of total weight loss at one to 2 years postoperatively, can regain an average of 7% of their total body weight from their lowest postoperative weight over the course of 10 years [6–7, 9, 19, 20]. According to those studies, the estimated average WR is about 15% (between 2 and 5% of weight from their lowest reported postoperative nadir weight) within 2 years after Roux en Y Gastric bypass. Those studies have reported an increase to 70% of patients between 2 and 5 years after Sleeve Gastrectomy, and 85% increase of WR at over 5 years post-surgery [10, 21] after that procedure. The high prevalence of weight regain after B/MS has resulted in a significant increase in revisional bariatric surgery [2, 6], which is a cause for increase in surgical risk and adverse outcomes to the patient [22, 23]. Causes of WR following B/MS are multifactorial and can be categorized into patient and surgical-specific causes. The summary of all aforementioned factors could outline the importance of following about weight regain:

1. Gastrointestinal, hormonal, and genetics factors
2. Gender, ethnic, and racial factors

3. Behavioral, dietary, lifestyle, and psychological factors

4. Performed Weight loss procedure as a technique and individual needs of the patient.

4. Gastrointestinal, hormonal, and Genetics factors for weight regain

There are known more than 30 gut hormone genes expressed and more than 100 bioactive peptides distributed in the gastrointestinal tract, which makes it the largest endocrine organ in the body [15, 17]. Several hormones in Gastrointestinal tract, which contribute to increase or decrease of food intake and in experimental studies, are directly associated with nutrition and body weight. That is the family of so-called PP-Fold Proteins. They consist of neuropeptide Y (NPY), peptide YY (PYY), and pancreatic polypeptide (PP). PYY and PP are secreted from gastrointestinal tract, whereas NPY is predominantly distributed within central nervous system [23]. Circulating PYY concentrations are low in fasted state and rise rapidly following a meal with a peak at 1–2 hours and remain elevated for several hours [24]. In both lean and obese humans, intravenous injection of PYY reduces appetite and food intake, suggesting that, unlike leptin, the sensitivity of PYY is preserved in obese subjects. Pancreatic Polypeptide (PP). PP is secreted from PP cells in the pancreatic islets of Langerhans. The anorectic effects of PP have been demonstrated in several experimental models. In leptin-deficient mice, repeated intraperitoneal injection of PP decreases body weight gain and ameliorates insulin resistance and hyperlipidemia [15]. GLP-1R is widely distributed particularly in the brain, GI tract, and pancreas [10]. It is known from experimental studies that circulating GLP-1 levels rise after a meal and fall in the fasted state. GLP-1 is associated with reduced food intake, and it can suppress glucagon secretion, leading to delayed gastric emptying [21]. Clinical trials in normal weight and obese subjects have also shown a reduction of food intake after a dose-dependent intravenous infusion of GLP-1. It is also known that Morbid obese patients have a blunted postprandial GLP-1 response compared to normal weight patients. GLP-1 is investigated about its potent incretin effect in addition to its anorectic action. That means that it can stimulate insulin secretion in a glucose-dependent manner following ingestion of carbohydrate. Experimental studies about application of Ozempic in clinical practice have confirmed positive effect of continuous subcutaneous infusion of GLP-1 to patients with type 2 diabetes for 6 weeks. GLP-1 infusion reduces appetite, body weight and improves glycemic control [25]. Research studies about the effect of Ozempic and Trulicity as Once-weekly subcutaneous injection have demonstrated greater improvements in glycemic control and weight loss in patients with Diabetes type 2 (DT2) and Obesity. On the other hand, Ghrelin is the only known orexigenic gut hormone involved in the mechanism of Morbid Obesity. Levels of circulating ghrelin increase before meal and fall rapidly in after meal period [25]. Fasting plasma levels of ghrelin are high in patients with anorexia nervosa [21] and in subjects with diet-induced weight loss. By contrast, obese patients have a less marked drop in plasma ghrelin after meal injection [25]. Dysregulation of ghrelin secretion is also implicated in the mechanism through which sleep disturbance contributes to Obesity. Subjects with short sleep duration have elevated ghrelin levels, reduced leptin, and high Body Mass Index (BMI) compared with patients with normal BMI and normal sleep duration [21].

Some authors as De Silva et al. [15] have investigated the brain function of obese patients during exposure to food pictures and intravenous infusion of Ghrelin with so-called functional magnetic resonance imaging. The investigations have revealed increased activation in the amygdala, orbitofrontal cortex, anterior insula, and striatum Furthermore, there are hypotheses that suggest that effects of ghrelin on the response of amygdala and orbitofrontal cortex are correlated with self-rated hunger ratings. Cholecystokinin (CCK) is another known gut hormone, which plays a role in food intake [25]. The experimental model confirms that CCK is secreted postprandially by the I cell of the small intestine into circulation, and it has a short plasma half-life of a few minutes. The investigations and studies into the function of Gastrointestinal hormones reveal that they play a significant role as mediators and triggering factors of weight regain in each patient. The process of investigation and adaptation of appropriate laboratory or Clinical tests to confirm that in clinical practice is too far now! However, the understanding and knowledge about secretion and expression of Gastrointestinal hormones can give us the basic selection criteria of Bariatric/Metabolic procedures in candidates of weight loss surgery and predict the long-term results of achieved or expected weight loss or weight regain.

The weight loss response after B/MS varies widely between individuals [6]. A part of this variation is probably due to genetic factors, as close biological relatives tend to have quite similar responses to weight loss interventions [19]. Several studies have tried with limited success to explore the significance of potential specific genetic determinants of the individual variation in weight loss after B/MS [2, 4, 5, 7, 8]. Reported studies of patients undergoing weight loss surgery have also pointed out a relationship between weight loss and genetic markers, associated with abdominal obesity. Anatomy and physiology of human body are individual; however, the polymorphisms of body fat distribution have been suggested to control the growth of human adipose tissue in three main pathways. The first one is so-called Adipogenesis. The second one is known as angiogenesis, and the third one is named as non-specified transcriptional regulation [26]. The first two pathways are responsible for adipose tissue function and expansion. The impairment of those two mechanisms can lead to metabolic disturbances through induction of hypoxia, inflammation, and fibrosis in the tissue [10]. The effects of fibrosis and reduced angiogenesis in adipose tissue are alerting factors for organ dysfunction in Morbid obese patients. Furthermore, fibrosis of adipose tissue may attenuate weight loss response after gastric bypass [1, 27]. Several hypotheses suggest that various genetic factors determinant for abdominal obesity and for weight loss responsiveness following surgical interventions may work via common pathways in adipogenesis and angiogenesis. One study has revealed that the association between Genetic Risk Score (GRS) and weight loss response to B/MS might be explained by the association between specific genetic markers and baseline anthropometrics, especially BMI [28]. Baseline BMI is known as a predicting factor for response to weight loss interventions. The choice of weight loss phenotype is therefore of great importance in this type of studies, investigating the association of weight loss and weight regain due to Genetic Factors. The same authors suggest that for mathematical reasons, the achieved BMI and excess weight loss variables are inversely associated with baseline BMI in B/MS cohorts [28]. Angiogenesis may be one of the mechanisms that govern the individual variation in response to weight loss treatment by possibly affecting adipose tissue flexibility.

Those studies open new horizons for surgical management of Morbid Obesity in patients with lower BMI but significant abdominal obesity and adipose tissue there. The studies also give the possibility to predict which procedures are most appropriate in such patients and what is the risk of WR on a long-term basis.

5. Gender, ethnic, and racial factors for weight regain after bariatric/metabolic surgery

Despite the overall success of bariatric surgery, weight loss and comorbidity remission appear to vary considerably across patients and procedures [2, 4, 5, 7, 8, 19, 29, 30]. Several studies, including a recent meta-analysis [31], have suggested that race is an important factor associated with weight loss and possibly comorbidity remission after BS [14, 24]. However, many of those reports represent single-center series with small numbers of patients. Furthermore, few of those studies have Data on the procedures such as: Sleeve Gastrectomy, Roux en Y Gastric bypass or one anastomosis Gastric bypass, comorbidity remission, or the effect of other socioeconomic variables.

The different aspects of social environment in Morbid Obese patients may also contribute to outcome after B/MS. Some studies have made efforts to allocate the spatial distribution of fast-food restaurants and supermarkets in connection to the residence of patients who have had weight loss surgery. The main conclusion of those studies is that access to foods meeting recommended dietary standards is an independent indicator for WR. They have also revealed a race difference despite the incomes of the population. Areas, predominantly inhabited by black people, regardless of income, have not had an adequate access to good-quality foods, compared to predominantly white, higher-income communities [32]. The infrastructure of the urban or non-urban areas also appears to contribute to the spread of Morbid Obesity in different living environments as indicator for WR. Transport links for commuters and access to nearby recreation centers are also contributing benchmarks, which can predict weight regain after B/MS. Lack of such facilities and transportation is isolating patients after surgery of effective postoperative follow-up and access to healthy lifestyle environment. There are also racial differences in understanding of good-looking body size. Review of surveys for body size outlines the prevalence of white obese women, who are looking for options of weight loss surgery or Gastric bypass due to impairment in quality of life, despite having lower body mass index values than the other race and sex groups [23]. The black men with Morbid Obesity are on the other pole of those surveys—they have the least social impairment with Obesity. The summary of those surveys reveals that ideal body size for themselves and the opposite sex are larger for black individuals than for white individuals [26, 33]. Morbid obese individuals in the black population have less social pressure to lose weight, but they can have pressure to lose less weight after B/MS by relatives and community [23]. Discrepancy between achieved and expected weight loss is the most listed common reason for dissatisfaction with surgery for both black patients (84%) and white patients (76%). The suggestion is that it might happen when there is patient–clinician discordance in racial identity [34]. Goleman et al. have revealed in their study that: "Gender and racial/ethnic background predict weight loss after Roux-en-Y gastric bypass independent of health and lifestyle behaviors" [35]. According to the authors: "non-Hispanic black men had significantly greater weight loss compared to non-Hispanic white men ($p < .05$)." The opposite, other studies do not reveal any difference in weight outcome between racial/ethnic groups of women, living in one and the same area. It means that socioeconomic factors and eating behaviors are more important predicting factors for WR than race and sex. However, it is known that patients with B/MS, who drink more diet soda than mineral water, have a higher percent of WR after surgery, independently of health status and lifestyle behaviors, age, and weight at the time of surgery. Another study has shown that blacks but not Hispanics have had a lower %EWL, compared to whites at 6 months after weight loss surgery. An interesting finding is that blacks have had a lower %EWL than Hispanics at every time point during the follow-up of patients [20]. The weight regain among different races varies, and it is evident even from the criteria for Bariatric/Metabolic Surgery in Europe, Asia, and the United States about BMI. Data suggest that there are significant differences in the prevalence of weight regain among patients post B/MS on different continents. Some of the published longest follow-up reviews have shown mean weight regain of about 4% after Roux-en-Y gastric bypass (RYGB) 3–7 years after surgery [32]. It contrasts with other studies, predominantly from Europe, which have reported that every fourth patient after RYGB or Sleeve Gastrectomy surgery can regain more than 15% of their body weight 5 years after the primary procedure [4, 5, 14]. It is also well-known that Asians are more prone to Diabetes Mellitus than white people with the same degree of BMI. Interestingly, there are significant differences in the algorithm for weight loss surgery in Asia and Europe, for example. The inclusion criteria for B/MS in Asia are lower with 2.5 kg/m^2 in each category of BMI. Surgery is also highly recommended for patients with Diabetes type 2 and cutoff BMI of 37.5 kg/m^2 compared to BMI over 40.0 kg/m^2 in Europe. The recommendations in Asia for Metabolic surgery suggest that patients with DT2 and BMI between 32.5 and 37.0 kg/m^2 should also be considered as candidates for Metabolic surgery, if their DT2 is poorly controlled. The review of data suggests that Asian patients will have lower WR up to 5 years after surgery due to lower threshold inclusion criteria for surgery as lower BMI. Because of differences in the baseline body height and weight, and body composition, it is not completely grounded to interpret the weight loss on the Asian communities according to Westerner physical standards. That is another evidence that WR on different continents and in different races is variable and individual approach and assessment of patients before or after BS are mandatory. The gender of the patient is another main contributing factor for WR after Bariatric/Metabolic Surgery. Several meta-analyses have revealed higher relative weight loss in men compared to women. Weight loss surgical outcome appears to be in favor of WL in men. That conclusion is based on data from two meta-analyses. Our experience can confirm the results of the one of those meta-analyses that female Obese patients are twice more likely to investigate and seek ways to lose weight than male patients. However, male patients can lose effectively more weight than female patients, and it can be up to 40% more likely successful [10]. There is a discrepancy on studies about influence of gender on weight loss and WR after B/MS. Some of them highlight male gender as an independent factor. On the other hand, other studies emphasize the role of exercise, diet, and eating behaviors as important factors for induced weight loss and deny the role of gender as indicator for WR [10, 36]. We are in favor of the second group of studies, because literature review of outcome after Bariatric/Metabolic Surgery in English and German language has shown no distinct difference in gender. That criterion is not reliable to give a definite answer, if a male or a female Morbid Obese patient with one and the same BMI is a better candidate for any weight loss procedure. Those six studies [37–42], which have detected better outcomes for male patients B/MS, are probably focused on gender mostly, rather than of type of procedure, BMI at time of surgery, and type of the procedure. It is known that female patients are seeking more often Sleeve Gastrectomy as option for weight loss or even Gastric Balloon. Male patients, due to higher BMI, are probably more open to Gastric bypass options than to Gastric Balloons or Sleeve Gastrectomy. The dilemma with gender is observed in the reviewed nonsurgical studies about the association between weight loss and gender. We have found 16 studies, which report no gender differences. The opposite, another 16 studies have pointed better weight loss in men compared to women. Unfortunately, most of the reviewed studies report gender difference in absolute weight loss. Although, it is known that relative weight loss is a more accurate criterion of measurement about detecting gender differences. Overall, systematic reviews confirm that women more likely not to achieve better weight loss than men. We have a worse situation, looking at studies and reports for WR after B/MS. The data are less conclusive about gender difference as predicting factor for WR. Most of all reviewed studies, mentioning WR, are in favor of no gender difference. There are three studies that have reported less WR in men, and other two studies have reported better weight loss maintenance in women. We would suggest that mandatory next step is to be initiated a conduct in Europe, Asia, and America with focus on gender differences in weight loss and WR, in particular to provide additional information and knowledge about potential reasons and solutions for treatment outcome in female and male bariatric patients.

6. Behavioral, dietary, lifestyle, and psychological factors

According to different authors [10, 23, 36, 43], there are four eating and lifestyle habits, independently associated with greater probability of post-surgical WR - **Table 1**. Those four types of post-bariatric surgery patients are called: a "sweet-eater," a "grazer," lifestyle habit as sedentarism, and patients consuming more daily calories or alcohol. A "sweet-eater" is someone who eats 50% or more of carbohydrates or consumes only simple carbohydrates. A "night eater" is defined as someone who three or more times per week consumes ≥50% of daily calories after 7 PM, who had difficulty sleeping, and who reports not being hungry at breakfast. Alcohol consumption is important and has been determined as independent factor for weight regain. Those patients are categorized in two groups: those drinking alcohol ≥2 times per week vs < 2 times per week. Sedentarism as definition describes the habits related to an inactive lifestyle, which can cause health problems such as Obesity in some people. There is another disorder, known as Binge eating Disorder (BED). That type of disorder led to implementation of one anastomosis Gastric bypass in Asia first and then on other continents, and it is associated with food culture of population in different countries. One of the definitions of BED describes it as eating substantially large amounts of food within short periods of time, accompanied by a sense of loss of control and feelings of disgust, guilt, and/or depression after binge episodes [34]. Approval of one anastomosis gastric bypass as accepted by IFSO standard weight loss surgical procedure significantly increased the number of patients with binge food disorders as candidates for B/MS. Their number varies from 10 to 40% according to available published officially results on Bariatric Registers. However, that inclusion criterion did not increase or propose an algorithm for a robust pre-operative investigation of those patients or adequate screening results for outcome after bariatric surgery. Therefore, we "branded" a proportionally huge number of

Type of eating disorder	A "sweet-eater"	Grazer	Sedentarism	Night eater
Definition	Someone, who eats 50% or more of carbohydrates or consumes only simple carbohydrates	Eating frequently at irregular intervals' – not quite the same as snacking, but probably more frequent.	The habits related to an inactive lifestyle which can cause health problems	Someone, who 3 or more times per week consumes ≥50% of daily calories after 7 PM, who had difficulty sleeping and who reports not being hungry at breakfast.
Psychological Factors	Depression and anxiety, self esteem	Triggered by stress, boredom, and emotional distress and worsens with "mindless eating" while watching television, surfing the internet, attending social meetings, or working in foodservice settings.	Generally inactive with mental and health problems, family history psychological disorders	Sleeping disorders, alcohol problems, depression, anxiety
Weight regain after B/M Surgery	Regain of 10–25% of EWL	Regain of 45–60% of EWL	Regain of 25–30% of EWL	Regain of 15–40% of EWL

Table 1.
Morbid obese patients with known eating and lifestyle habits and WR.

patients as those with "binge food disorder," who qualify for a weight loss procedure. But those patients aren't diagnosed or treated for BED before surgery. They probably have certain aspects of the disorder (e.g., loss of control about food and eating), and they may emerge post-surgery, potentially resulting in negative long-term weight loss outcomes or weight regain [36]. The conclusion is that we need beforehand preoperative assessment of patients with BED by experienced behavioral health professionals. The process of diagnosis and management of patients with BED, candidates for B/MS is critical, as the underlying dynamics of the disorder usually will persist after surgery [27]. Effective treatment for BED or maladaptive eating before surgery potentially will predict outcome of surgery. Such treatment will help the patient to cope successfully with depression, anxiety, or trauma after weight loss surgery. The process of long-term management must include nutrition counseling, medical care, and follow-up to 5 years after surgery. Outcome of patient's treatment as individual or in a group with similar patients plus involvement of family therapy is a significant predicting factor for WR after one anastomosis gastric bypass [44]. The absence of such a multidisciplinary approach to treatment is a potential risk for the eating disorder to persist or morph into another form of eating disorder as grazing. According to most definitions, available on Intranet, "grazer" is a person who eats snacks or small food portions several times a day, without consuming a primary meal. Grazing is a more serious behavioral health disorder, as it can develop a higher risk of vomiting and gastrointestinal symptoms. According to some Bariatric surgeons, dysphagia and dumping after weight loss surgery can teach the patients to change their eating habits. Unfortunately, that statement is wrong. Regular vomiting postoperatively can cause nutritional deficiencies, dental caries, esophagitis, and gastric ulcers, all of which can further impact food choices and intake [43]. The misperception among some patients that frequent vomiting helps to prevent WR should be corrected and noticed by responsible Dietitian and surgeon on follow-up clinic reviews immediately and negative effects of the condition to be explained and treated accordingly. Even patients who lack a formally diagnosed eating disorder can lose control over their eating habits after B/MS and that loss of control might increase around the 2-year point [26, 33]. Literature review confirms that loss of control overeating or appearance of grazing after surgery is associated with less excess weight loss, greater WR, and decreased perceived quality of life [23]. It is known that patients who engage in grazing behaviors two or fewer times per week after surgery have poorer percentage of excess weight loss and larger weight regain than those who had not has such a problem.

There are also so-called: "Other Maladaptive Eating Behaviors." Dietitians and Nutritional specialists have found that maladaptive eating behaviors may also develop in some patients. It is explained that attempts to avoid vomiting after B/MS are linked to the development of food aversion, protein malnutrition, and micronutrient deficiencies. Unfortunately, those maladaptive disorders also influence long-term weight loss outcomes and quality of life [45]. There is another group of patients with eating disorders. They generally avoid solid foods and eat softer, high-calorie foods such as chocolate, candy, and ice cream. The consumption of excess calories, particularly from refined carbohydrates and saturated fats, is another objective predictor of WR in such patients. Maladaptive eaters among patients with weight loss surgery consider easier to swallow soups, crackers, and cheese than solid foods. Overconsumption of softer, calorie-dense foods ("soft food syndrome") provides inadequate nutrition and decreased satiety. Another condition, which ultimately contributes to excessive energy intake and weight gain. There is also another group of patients who prefer fully to engage in restrictive model of eating, failing to consume adequate calories due to an intense fear of stretching the stomach pouch and regaining weight. There is a psychological factor in those patients: preoccupation with weight and body image, but that condition can lead to macro- and micronutrient deficiencies and eventual WR [33]. Bariatric surgery developed another restrictive eating disorder. It is known as: "post-surgical eating avoidance disorder" or PSEAD. The disorder is described as eating very little to avoid WR or experience of an almost "phobic" reaction to food. Healthful eating habits should be reinforced months before surgery. Active role of Dietitian and engagement of patient are mandatory to prevent the onset of maladaptive eating patterns, gastrointestinal distress, and WR. The Dietitian should be certain that candidates for weight loss surgery have made significant behavioral changes involving nutrition and food as eating slowly and exercising portion control. The use of cognitive behavioral strategies to encourage mindful eating and appropriate food choices is another successful part of the game about the process of teaching [26]. The regular follow-up from multidisciplinary team members will recognize early maladaptive eating behaviors or food aversions, expressed by patient, and will encourage him to maintain adequate lifelong nutrition, and not rely on BS alone to improve their weight loss outcomes and health benefits. The early changes in total energy intake and macronutrient composition during the first 6 months after surgery are found to be a predictor of long-term success with 10 years follow-up [21, 25]. Data confirm that eating 100 additional daily calories is associated with a 30% increase in odds of WR 3–4 years after BS.

It is known that preoperative physical activity levels and eating style do not correlate with maximum weight loss. However, there is a negative correlation between preoperative physical activity levels and external eating and a positive correlation between physical activity levels and restrained eating [22]. According to a paper, presented at IFSO 22nd World Congress; August 29–September 2, 2017, in London: "There was a less weight regain in patients who reported more [physical activity] after RYGB. Eating style does not seem to affect weight regain" [3]. A study from 2021 confirms that low level of physical activity and longer sedentary time have occurred more frequently in those with high WR and longer time since weight loss surgery [28]. Mental health conditions are common among bariatric surgery patients. Abnormal eating patterns, binge eating disorder in particular: depression, alcohol and drug addiction are reported as predictive factors of weight regain after BS [23, 24]. Psychological assessment and identification of those patients preoperatively are a major contributing factor for good long-term results after Bariatric/Metabolic Surgery. Unfortunately, the limitations of funding for weight loss surgery and the whole process of preparation of a patient for such type of treatment are an ongoing problem in Europe and all over the world. Patients who choose BS must be educated to understand that Obesity is a chronic disease! Bariatric/Metabolic surgery is only one of the tools, which can effectively help the patient to achieve significant weight loss, but inadequate postoperative adherence to recommendations can override that tools' efficacy, leading to weight regain.

7. Weight loss procedure as a technique and selection of type of operation as a factor for weight regain after bariatric surgery

The data review of different search engines about WR after well-known weight loss procedures worldwide is presented in **Table 2**. The data represent current estimated success of those procedures on a long-term follow-up. However, they do not represent the spread of different procedures and their popularity around the globe.

Sleeve Gastrectomy is the most common weight loss procedure all over the world so far. Its prevalence in United States and parts of Asia can be explained with eating habits or preferences of the patients there. For example, India's population is more than 50% vegetarian. Malabsorptive procedures such as Roux en Y or one anastomosis Gastric bypass have significant side effects on vegetarian patients and they struggle to compensate their protein and nutrient balance. So, the practice and experience reversed the type of weight loss procedures to Sleeve Gastrectomy (SLG) there. The growing number of weight loss operations all over the world, according to IFSO survey in 2016 total number of procedure, was 700,000 [46], provide enormous data about Bariatric procedures and patients. However, weight regain after bariatric surgery is one of the related topics with a relatively limited number of publications [47]. Long-term results of bariatric patient series reveal that after 2 years postoperatively, patients' rate of losing weight tends to decelerate [48]. Despite those results, Sleeve Gastrectomy is still the preferable operation for weight loss for patients and surgeons around the world. The numbers of Sleeve procedures are significantly higher than bypass procedures, according to data from IFSO Register and explanations of that status are not associated with long-term outcome

Type of procedure	WR after 2 years	WR after 3 years	WR after 4 years	WR after 5 years	WR after 10 years
Lap band procedure	5% with >20% of EWL	25% with >50% of EWL	38% with >40% of EWL	Over 60% regained >50% of EWL	No data, most bands removed
Sleeve gastrectomy	2% with up to 5% of EWL	12% with >20% of EWL	18% with >35% of EWL	25% with >40% of EWL	40% with >40% of EWL
Roux en Y gastric bypass	1% with up to 5% of EWL	2% with up to 5% of EWL	3.5% with 10% of EWL	3.9 to 4.0% >10% of EWL	4.5% >10% of EWL
One anastomosis gastric bypass	0.2% with up to 5% of EWL	1.0% with up to 5% of EWL	3.0% with up to 5% of EWL	3.5% with >10% of EWL	5% with >5% of EWL
Duodenal switch	0%	0.8% with up to 2% of EWL	1.5% with up to 5% of EWL	2.0% with >5% of EWL	2.5% with >5% of EWL

Table 2.
Weight regain due to type of weight loss procedure: (electronic database data, including PubMed, MEDLINE, Embase, CINAHL, Web of Science and Scopus).

and probability for WR [22]. Long-term results have shown that Sleeve Gastrectomy procedure is associated with significant WR within 10 years after surgery. The other main problem with that weight loss procedure is about development of a restrictive eating pattern and intractable gastroesophageal reflux, requiring revisional surgery in up to 20% of patients after primary procedure. The aspects of weight regain after SLG have been discussed in several publications; however, there are no systematic reviews, encompassing all surgical issues about the procedure. Anatomical/surgical factors of weight regain after LSG are identified as: an initial large sleeve, incompletely resected fundus, and a large remnant antrum. We think there are three other issues about WR after Sleeve Gastrectomy as a technique and patient selection: Medical tourism as a factor for spread of the procedure, applicable to different Body Mass Index, even in super Obese patients as a first-stage procedure, the growing number of weight loss procedures performed privately, rather than in public Hospitals. The use of different bougies or dissection of the stomach to 2 or 4 cm above the pylorus has been investigated, and there are no standards about impact of that on weight regain. Several studies have showed no difference in dissection of the antrum as a predicting factor for weight regain after SLG. The learning curve of the surgeon and dissection around the short gastric vessels and left crura are also factors contributing to WR after LSG, according to different studies [2, 4, 5, 7, 8, 49, 50]. Medical tourism and offer of the SLG in private are another contributing factor for WR. Interestingly, there is a growing amount of data for patients, admitted to UK NHS hospitals in emergency after SLG abroad. One such example is about a case of our practice: a 45-year-old lady, who had a SLG in Turkey. She has developed bleeding from staple line, she has been transfused with 2 Units of blood there and sent home back on a commercial flight. The lady has been admitted from Airport to our Hospital with a HB of 89.0 g/l and urgent CT scan showed a big hematoma around the greater curvature of the stomach and spleen. Her management has been conservative, and outcome has been uneventful. However, she has been followed for 6 months only after surgery and her BMI at time of admission was 52.0. There are several other reports for admission of patients 1–2 weeks after SLG abroad, due to severe nausea, vomiting, or even dehydration and motility problems. It is known that about 15% of population in the United Kingdom has motility disorders of the esophagus. As we mentioned above, those disorders plus reflux after SLG are important factors for WR in those patients. The robust pre-operative investigations of bariatric patients and selection of the appropriate type of weight loss procedure are the key for long-term good results and prevention of substantial WR. Unfortunately, the economy recession and restrictions of funding about weight loss surgery are a serious concern about the increase of Bariatric procedures in NHS and the right of more Morbid Obese patients to have a proper selection and access to weight loss surgery. The other main issue is that in some parts of the United Kingdom, the only offered bariatric surgery in NHS is the Sleeve Gastrectomy. The patients with BMI over 50.0 are struggling to get an access for a bypass procedure, funded by NHS, in another Bariatric Center due to administrative problems. Weight regain after Roux en Y or one anastomosis Gastric bypass is also reported and documented. The WR after those two procedures is less than SLG, and the main reasons are associated with the volume and shape of the Gastric pouch, the diameter of gastro-jejunal anastomosis, and the length of biliary limb. The Surgeon, who first proposed mini-gastric bypass–Rutledge, describes his vision that dumping, as outcome of the procedure, contributes significantly to weight loss after surgery. Unfortunately, the motility of esophagus as a factor for WR after mini or one anastomosis gastric bypass is not investigated robustly so far. The quick transit of food from esophagus to stomach can accelerate appearance of eating disorders and minimize the effect of restriction. Most of the experts in bariatric surgery recommend the pouch-jejunal anastomosis not to be created immediately under esophago-gastric junction as the pouch will not be functioning optimally in terms of weight loss and long results can be disappointing. They also recommend the anastomosis between the pouch and jejunum to be on the side of the greater curvature and a length of 2–4 cm of the lesser curve of the stomach to be incorporated in the pouch.

It is known that Poiseuille's Law in physics postulates that the flow rate through a tube is inversely proportional to its length. Slow flow or emptying of the pouch is desirable after gastric bypass and contributes to the restriction [45, 51]. According to that law seems that the shape (length and diameter) may be rather more important than the size itself [52]. Another law in physics, known as LaPlace Law, postulates that the pressure required to distend a structure (tube) is inversely proportional to its radius. Interestingly, those two laws in physics have their application in creation of gastric pouch during bypass surgery. The shape and form of the pouch plus diameter of anastomosis with jejunum are mandatory for the optimal function of the gastric bypass. Literature review has confirmed that longer and narrower gastric pouch has a less dilatation in time after gastric bypass surgery. It combines slower emptying of the pouch, less probability for dumping syndrome, and less stretching 2 years after surgery. The Fobi Pouch Gastric bypass is an example for such a gastric pouch; however, evidence of long-term results is necessary to completely implement the postulate of the mentioned above physics law in Bariatric surgical practice [50]. WR, which is seen 3–5 years following laparoscopic gastric bypass surgery, is often explained because of enlargement of the pouch [22]. For durable restriction and therefore weight loss, a long narrow pouch is recommended. The length of pouch after one anastomosis gastric bypass (OAGB) is important about bile reflux and its complication also can contribute to WR.

There are still many debates about postoperative bile reflux after mini or one anastomosis gastric bypass and its significance about quality of life of patients and WR. The accepted standard in the technique is length of the sleeve—more than 16 cm. However, there are also different "tips" for avoiding the bile reflux and hence weight regain 5 years after the procedure. There are no statistically significant data to confirm the importance of the proposed "tips." The BMI over 50.0 kg/m^2 before surgery, age of the patient at time of surgery, concurrent eating and metabolic disorders, length of the biliary limb, and diameter of the anastomosis are probably the predicting factors for outcome and WR after gastric bypass surgery [51, 53]. Innovations and suggestions as Fundo-Ring OAGB, wherein one anastomosis gastric bypass the proximal part of the pouch is wrapped with a fundus of the excluded part of the stomach to treat bile reflux and WR, are promising and interesting. However, long-term results are needed. The banding of Gastric pouch or the Gastric Sleeve with Fobi ring is another promising technique for surgical management of weight regain, and the long-term results will reveal more detailed information about feasibility and effectiveness of that proposed technique. The size of gastro-jejunal anastomosis is another important factor for WR. The recommendations are about a diameter of the anastomosis of 1.5–2.0 cm. Unfortunately, such diameter of anastomosis is a significant problem in the United Kingdom, whereas patients have esophageal dysmotility problems and their eating habits are different of those in patients from Europe and Middle East. Due to prevention of early complications with stricture and vomiting after Roux en Y Gastric bypass surgery, most Bariatric Centers in the United Kingdom prefer to do a stapled gastro-jejunal anastomosis with 45 mm reload. The short-term results and outcome of those patients are excellent; however, about 40% of them have a risk to develop significant WR 3–5 years after surgery. Unfortunately, the International Bariatric Registers are not giving adequate and exact information about the association between WR and the diameter of Gastro-jejunal anastomosis. Endoscopic management of the gastro-jejunal anastomosis as a size is effective and safe option in experienced hands as a first step for management of WR after Roux en Y Gastric bypass [54]. It allows several attempts in first instance to treat wide anastomosis or even peptic ulcers and is highly recommended opposite revisional surgery for management of WR in high-volume centers [51].

The length of biliary-pancreatic limb (BPL) has been the subject of several investigations about its effect on weight loss and hence WR after Gastric bypass surgery. The distalization of the biliopancreatic limb is associated with greater weight loss even in revisional surgery. The suggestion is based on data that patients with short biliary limb—between 50 and 60 cm, achieve less weight loss and regain a higher percentage of EXL within 5 years after surgery [14, 35]. However, the lessons of human anatomy should not be forgotten. The length of a small bowel in a human body is proportional to his height. The longer biliary limb in a bariatric patient postulates measurement of total small bowel length or at least of the common channel in order to avoid serious postoperative complications such as protein malnutrition and diarrhea [40, 55]. A study from the USA describes a racial difference in patients with distal biliary limb. According to Khattab et al. [34], patients with Afro-American and Asian origin do not tolerate the distal gastric bypass as well as white patients. There are other authors, who have several arguments toward the significance of the biliary limb length [35]. They think that reduction of common channel length should be tailored individually and there are other concomitant factors, which are responsible for weight loss and WR in every patient [35]. That factor, plus discrepancies in small bowel measurement during surgery, can play a significant role in mechanisms of weight regain after B/M Surgery.

Several experimental studies have tried to interpret the presence of undiluted bile acids in the distal small bowel. They suggest that there are specific receptors, which are triggered by undiluted bile acids in the L cells in ileum, and those cells are responsible for enhanced release of GLP-1 and PYY hormones in the small bowel. Their theory explains why serum bile acid concentration is after Roux en Y Gastric bypass and that can lead to increased energy expenditure [17, 51]. Modern theories about better weight loss after malabsorptive procedures are based on hormonal mechanisms and interactions, which at the end achieve lower HbA1C levels, found among the group with longer biliary limb. Therefore, nutritional disturbances are more pronounced, and the diarrhea score significantly increased in the longer BPL group due to eating habits of the patient [24]. It is likely that these side effects will be observed in future reports on the patients with a longer BPL. So, the BPL length as a factor for WR is still in debate, and more randomized and long-term studies are required to obtain medical-based evidence for importance and influence of BPL over WR after Roux en Y Gastric bypass or one anastomosis bypass surgery. The length of BPL is in direct correlation with BMI of the patient nowadays. The standard length of BPL is 100 cm in length in patients with BMI between 40.0 and 48.0. When BMI is more than 48.0 and height of the patient is over 170 cm, BPL length is recommended to be 120–150 cm in length and the patient to have a common channel at least of 250 cm to avoid severe malnutrition, diarrhea, and vitamin deficiency.

Bariatric/Metabolic procedures, proposed for management of WR as SADI-S procedure, biliopancreatic diversion, and duodenal switch have been well investigated and documented, and their routine use has been largely abandoned due to abovementioned possibilities for complications and nutritional problems. Those patients need very close review and support by specialized Clinics and Hospitals for management of such nutritional and malabsorptive issues more than 2 years after primary procedure. However, the data of medical-based evidence and Guidelines of Bariatric Surgical Societies around the world are in a discrepancy about follow-up of patients after weight loss surgery. Data suggest that all B/MS patients to be reviewed and followed almost 5 years after surgery, but Guidelines recommend a cutoff up to 2 years after primary procedures, leaving a significant and not relevant burden of follow-up to General Practitioners.

8. Summary

Most Morbid obese patients emphasize on importance of having someone, who can give them support in a way that they have felt understood. Most of them also expect bariatric surgery to end their struggle with weight and eating [56]. Unfortunately, Bariatric patients are often unprepared for weight regain and react with emotional distress, i.e., hopelessness, discouragement, shame, and frustration. Regaining weight might be a devastating experience that contribute to a negative spiral in weight management. Negative self-image, maladaptive eating behaviors, substance's use, and overall impaired psychosocial functioning in turn have been associated with internalized weight bias and further weight management difficulties [10, 14, 23, 24, 26, 28, 33]. Postoperative alcohol use has been identified as a predictor for weight regain and even severe episodes of pancreatitis, which unfortunately caused death in two of our cases on 10 years' follow-up after BS. Addiction transfer refers to a shift, where food rewards are replaced

Psychological background of patient	Body Mass Index and waist circumference at time of surgery and	Race and social status	Is procedure relevant to BMI and co-morbidity	Post op support and follow up
Anxiety and depression not treated effectively before surgery	BMI over 50 or 55	Poor social status, Lives in a community, where obesity is not a health issue	Lap Band or Sleeve Gastrectomy in patients with BMI between 42 and 50	Surgery done privately
Eating and binge eating disorders	minimal or no weight loss before surgery	Female patients with Hispanic or Afro American origin	Anastomosis of more than 2.5 cm and larger pouch	No national system for regular follow up
Mobility and physical activity	<50% of required weight loss on second year after surgery	Lack of healthcare system for tackling of Obesity	Biliary limb less than 100 cm	Lack of Dietitian review in the first 3 years after surgery
Alcohol intake. Self-control and feeling of disgust	Waist circumference more than 115 cm in female patients	Family support and community support	History of DT2 and Sleep Apnoea more than 5 years	Lack of regular psychological support after surgery

Table 3.
Summarized predicting factors for weight regain.

with other substances post-surgically, which may also contribute to weight regain [24]. Procedures, perioperative protocols, and post operative management for bariatric surgery will evolve over time. Solution of those complex problems and management of WR require a longer follow-up and support of experienced multidisciplinary teams. Most of the contributing factors of WR are summarized on **Table 3**. However, the discussion for a funded and patient-oriented routine review by experts and specialists in Bariatric/Metabolic Surgery up to 5 years after the primary procedure is still open. We need a more serious and honest debate about extended funding of those activities by Governments and Health Insurance Funds.

Author details

Ivaylo Tzvetkov
Hospital Brain and Heart, Pleven, Bulgaria

*Address all correspondence to: tzvetkov62@gmail.com

References

[1] Adams TD, Davidson LE, Litwin SE, et al. Weight and metabolic outcomes 12 years after gastric bypass. The New England Journal of Medicine. 2017;**377**:1143-1155

[2] Sjöström L. Review of the key results from the Swedish Obese Subjects (SOS) trial—A prospective controlled intervention study of bariatric surgery. Journal of Internal Medicine. 2013;**273**(3):219-234

[3] Karlsson J, Taft C, Sjöström L, Torgerson JS, Sullivan M. Psychosocial functioning in the obese before and after weight reduction: construct validity and responsiveness of the obesity-related problems scale. International Journal of Obesity and Related Metabolic Disorders. 2003;**27**:617-663

[4] Peterli R, Steinert RE, Woelnerhanssen B, Peters T, ChristofelCourtin C, Gass M, et al. Metabolic and hormonal changes after laparoscopic Roux-en-Y gastric bypass and sleeve gastrectomy: A randomized, prospective trial. Obesity Surgery. 2012;**22**(5):740-801

[5] Varma S, Clark JM, Schweitzer M, Magnuson T, Brown TT, Lee CJ. Weight regain in patients with symptoms of post-bariatric surgery hypoglycemia. Surgery for Obesity and Related Diseases. 2017;**13**(10):1728-1734

[6] El Ansari W, Elhag W. Weight regain and insufficient weight loss after bariatric surgery: Defnitions, prevalence, mechanisms, predictors, prevention and management strategies, and knowledge gaps—A scoping review. Obesity Surgery. 2021;**31**(4):1755-1766

[7] Courcoulas AP, King WC, Belle SH, Berk P, Flum DR, Garcia L, et al. Seven-year weight trajectories and health outcomes in the Longitudinal Assessment of Bariatric Surgery (LABS) study. JAMA Surgery. 2018;**153**(5):427-434

[8] Mingrone G, Panunzi S, De Gaetano A, Guidone C, Iaconelli A, Nanni G, et al. Bariatric-metabolic surgery versus conventional medical treatment in obese patients with type 2 diabetes: 5-year follow-up of an open-label, single-centre, randomized controlled trial. Lancet. 2015;**386**(9997):964-973

[9] Brissman M, Beamish AJ, Olbers T, Marcus C. Prevalence of insufficient weight loss 5 years after Roux-en-Y gastric bypass: Metabolic consequences and prediction estimates: A prospective registry study. BMJ Open. 2021;**11**(3):e046407

[10] Kalarchian MA, Marcus MD. Psychosocial interventions pre and post bariatric surgery. European Eating Disorders Review. 2015;**23**(6):457-462

[11] Ahlman H, Nilsson: The gut as the largest endocrine organ in the body. Ann Oncol: 12 Suppl. 2001;2:S63-8 8. DOI: 10.1093

[12] Carvalho A Jr, Turato ER, Chaim EA, Magdaleno R Jr. Weight regain among women after metabolic and bariatric surgery: A qualitative study in Brazil. Trends in Psychiatry and Psychotherapy. 2014;**36**(3):140-146

[13] Jones L, Cleator J, Yorke J. Maintaining weight loss after bariatric surgery: When the spectator role is no longer enough. Clinical Obesity. 2016;**6**(4):249-258

[14] Santo MA, Riccioppo D, Pajecki D, Kawamoto F, de Cleva R, Antonangelo L,

et al. Weight regain after gastric bypass: Influence of gut hormones. Obesity Surgery. 2016;**26**(5):919-25

[15] Akila De Silva, Victoria Salem, Paul M. Matthews, Waljit S. Dhillo: The Use of Functional MRI to Study Appetite Control in the CNS, Exp Diabetes Res. 2012:764017. DOI: 10.1155/2012/764017

[16] Aliakbarian H, Bhutta HY, Heshmati K, et al. Pre-operative predictors of weight loss and weight regain following Roux-en-Y gastric bypass surgery: A prospective human study. Obesity Surgery. 2020;**30**:4852-4859

[17] Sarwer DB, Allison KC, Wadden TA, Ashare R, Spitzer JC, McCuen-Wurst C, et al. Psychopathology, disordered eating, and impulsivity as predictors of outcomes of bariatric surgery. Surgery for Obesity and Related Diseases. 2019;**15**(4):650-655

[18] Rudolph A, Hilbert A. Post-operative behavioral management in bariatric surgery: A systematic review and meta-analysis of randomized controlled trials. Obesity Reviews. 2013;**14**:292-302

[19] Hatoum IJ, Greenawalt DM, Cotsapas C, Reitman ML, Daly MJ, Kaplan LM. Heritability of the weight loss response to gastric bypass surgery. The Journal of Clinical Endocrinology and Metabolism. 2011;**96**(10):E1630-E1633

[20] Odom J, Zalesin KC, Washington TL, Miller WW, Hakmeh B, Zaremba DL, et al. Behavioral predictors of weight regain after bariatric surgery. Obesity Surgery. 2010;**20**(3):349-356

[21] Smith KE, Engel SG, Stefen KJ, Garcia L, Grothe K, Koball A, et al. Problematic alcohol use and associated characteristics following bariatric surgery. Obesity Surgery. 2018;**28**(5): 1248-1254

[22] Alexandrou P. Sakarellos Sp. Davakis M. Vailas,N. Dimitriu Al. Paralampros et al: Revision of Roux-en-Y gastric bypass for inadequate weight loss or weight regain, review article, In vivo. 2022;**36**(1):30-39. DOI: 10.21873/invivo.12673

[23] Bradley LE, Forman EM, Kerrigan SG, et al. A pilot study of an acceptance-based behavioural intervention for weight regain after bariatric surgery. Obesity Surgery. 2016;**26**:2433-2441

[24] Jacobsen SH, Olesen SC, Dirksen C, et al. Changes in gastrointestinal hormone responses, insulin sensitivity, and beta-cell function within 2 weeks after gastric bypass in non-diabetic subjects. Obesity Surgery. 2012;**22**:1084-1096

[25] King WC, Chen JY, Courcoulas AP, Dakin GF, Engel SG, Flum DR, et al. Alcohol and other substance use after bariatric surgery: Prospective evidence from a U.S. multicenter cohort study. Surgery for Obesity and Related Diseases. 2017;**13**(8):1392-1402

[26] Bradley LE, Forman EM, Kerrigan SG, Goldstein SP, Butryn ML, Thomas JG, et al. Project HELP: A remotely delivered behavioural intervention for weight regain after bariatric surgery. Obesity Surgery. 2017;**27**(3):586-598

[27] Dawes AJ, Maggard-Gibbons M, Maher AR, Booth MJ, MiakeLye I, Beroes JM, et al. Mental health conditions among patients seeking and undergoing bariatric surgery: A meta-analysis. Journal of the American Medical Association. 2016;**315**(2):150-163

[28] Cummings DE, Weigle DS, Frayo RS, et al. Plasma ghrelin levels after diet-induced weight loss or gastric bypass surgery. The New England Journal of Medicine. 2002;**346**:1623-1630

[29] Freire RH, Borges MC, Alvarez-Leite JI, Toulson Davisson Correia MI. Food quality, physical activity, and nutritional follow-up as determinant of weight regain after Roux-en-Y gastric bypass. Nutrition. 2012;**28**(1):53-58

[30] Karmali S, Brar B, Shi X, et al. Weight recidivism post-bariatric surgery: A systematic review. Obesity Surgery. 2013;**23**:1922-1933

[31] Kofman MD, Lent MR, Swencionis C. Maladaptive eating patterns, quality of life, and weight outcomes following gastric bypass: Results of an Internet survey. Obesity (Silver Spring). 2010;**18**(10):1938-1943

[32] Leonard K. Welsh, Andrew R Luhrs, Gerardo Davalos, Ramon Diaz, et al. Racial disparities in bariatric surgery complications and mortality using the MBSAQIP data registry. Obesity Surgery. 2020;**30**:3099-3110. DOI: 10.1007/s11695-020-04657-3

[33] Beck NN, Johannsen M, Støving RK, et al. Do postoperative psychotherapeutic interventions and support groups influence weight loss following bariatric surgery? A systematic review and meta-analysis of randomized and nonrandomized trials. Obesity Surgery. 2012;**22**:1790-1797

[34] Khattab MA, Mohammed ATA, Alqahtani AZM, Alqahtani EZM, Alslim MMA, Alharbi NEA, et al. The role of ethnic disparities in the outcomes of bariatric surgery: A systematic review and meta-analysis. Cureus; 14(5):e24743, doi: 10.7759/cureus.24743, 2022

[35] Karen J Coleman, John Brookey: Gender and racial/ethnic background predict weight loss after Roux-en-Y gastric bypass independent of health and lifestyle behaviors. Obesity Surgery. 2014;**24**(10):1729-1736. DOI: 10.1007/s11695-014-1268-0

[36] Faria SL, de Oliveira KE, Lins RD, Faria OP. Nutritional management of weight regain after bariatric surgery. Obesity Surgery. 2010;**20**(2):135-139

[37] Järvholm K, Olbers T, Engström M. Patients' views of long-term results of bariatric surgery for super-obesity: Sustained effects, but continuing struggles. Surgery for Obesity and Related Diseases. 2021;**17**(6):1152-1164

[38] Tolvanen L, Svensson Å, Hemmingsson E, Christenson A, Lagerros YT. Perceived and preferred social support in patients experiencing weight regain after bariatric surgery—A qualitative study. Obesity Surgery. 2021;**31**(3):1256-1264

[39] Ogden J, Clementi C, Aylwin S. The impact of obesity surgery and the paradox of control: A qualitative study. Psychology & Health. 2006;**21**(2):273-293

[40] Heinberg LJ, Bond DS, Carroll I, et al. Identifying mechanisms that predict weight trajectory after bariatric surgery: Rationale and design of the biobehavioral trial. Surgery for Obesity and Related Diseases. 2020;**16**:1816-1826

[41] Sugerman HJ, Kellum JM, DeMaria EJ. Conversion of proximal to distal gastric bypass for failed gastric bypass for superobesity. Journal of Gastrointestinal Surgery. 1997;**1**:517-524

[42] Lauti M, Kularatna M, Hill AG, MacCormick AD. Weight regain following sleeve gastrectomy—A systematic review. Obesity Surgery. 2016;**26**(6):1326-1334

[43] Koball AM, Ames G, Goetze RE. Addiction transfer and other behavioural changes following bariatric surgery. The Surgical Clinics of North America. 2021;**101**(2):323-333

[44] Groven KS, Glenn NM. The experience of regaining weight following weight loss surgery: A narrative-phenomenological exploration. Health Care for Women International. 2016;**37**(11):1185-1202

[45] Chansaenroj P, Aung L, Lee WJ, Chen SC, Chen JC, Ser KH. Revision procedures after failed adjustable gastric banding: Comparison of efficacy and safety. Obesity Surgery. 2017;**27**(11):2861-2867

[46] Yilmaz H, Ece I, Sahin M. Revisional surgery after failed laparoscopic sleeve gastrectomy: Retrospective analysis of causes, results, and technical considerations. Obesity Surgery. 2017;**27**(11):2855-2860

[47] Noel P, Nedelcu M, Eddbali I, Manos T, Gagner M. What are the long-term results 8 years after sleeve gastrectomy? Surgery for Obesity and Related Diseases. 2017;**13**(7):1110-1115

[48] Felsenreich DM, Langer FB, Kefurt R, et al. Weight loss, weight regain, and conversions to Roux-en-Y gastric bypass: 10-year results of laparoscopic sleeve gastrectomy. Surgery for Obesity and Related Diseases. 2016;**12**(9):1655-1662

[49] Rudolph A, Hilbert A. Post-operative behavioural management in bariatric surgery: A systematic review and meta-analysis of randomized controlled trials Review, Obes Rev. 2013;**14**(4):292-302. DOI: 10.1111/obr.12013

[50] Torres J. Why I prefer gastric bypass distal Roux-en-Y gastroileostomy. Obesity Surgery. 1991;**1**:189-194

[51] Stroh C, Weiner R, Wolff S, et al. Revisional surgery and reoperations in obesity and metabolic surgery: Data analysis of the German bariatric surgery registry 2005-2012. Der Chirurg. 2015;**86**(4):346-354

[52] Tran DD, Nwokeabia ID, Purnell S, Zafar SN, Ortega G, Hughes K, et al. Revision of Roux-en-Y gastric bypass for weight regain: A systematic review of techniques and outcomes. Obesity Surgery. 2016;**26**:1627-1634

[53] Sánchez-Pernaute A, Rubio MÁ, Conde M, Arrue E, Pérez-Aguirre E, Torres A. Single-anastomosis duodenoileal bypass as a second step after sleeve gastrectomy. Surgery for Obesity and Related Diseases. 2015;**11**(2):351-355

[54] Angrisani A, Santonicola PI, et al. Bariatric surgery and endoluminal procedures: 2017. IFSO worldwide survey 2014. Obesity Surgery. 2017;**27**(9):2279-2289

[55] Noun R, Zeidan S, Riachi E, Abboud B, Chalhoub V, Yazigi A. Mini-gastric bypass for revision of failed primary restrictive procedures: A valuable option. Obesity Surgery. 2007;**17**(5):684-688

[56] Karlsson J, Taft C, Sjöström L, Torgerson JS, Sullivan M. Psychosocial functioning in the obese before and after weight reduction: Construct validity and responsiveness of theobesity-related problems scale. International Journal of Obesity and Related Metabolic Disorders. 2003;**27**:617-663

Chapter 5

Long Term Success and Follow-Up after Bariatric Surgery

Juaquito M. Jorge and Frederick M. Tiesenga

Abstract

Obesity is a multifactorial, chronic, and progressive disease whose pathogenesis is tied to a strong genetic component as well as a multitude of hormonal, metabolic, psychological, cultural and behavioral factors. Understanding the role these factors play, screening for them, and managing them appropriately, is important for effective weight loss. Psychology and behavior have profound implications on a patient's willingness and ability to engage in treatment and to follow up after bariatric surgery. Dietary education, presence of clear expectations, patient adherence to recommendations, and follow-up, directly impact bariatric surgery outcomes. Understanding postsurgical outcome success and failure and identifying best clinical practices for optimizing and maintaining results after bariatric surgery continues to be a work in process.

Keywords: obesity, behavioral modification, dietary adherence, long-term follow-up, long-term success

1. Introduction

Obesity perception and management has undergone a paradigm shift in the last few decades. Our understanding of the complex factors and etiologies of obesity as a chronic illness, improvements in medical and surgical treatment options, and access to care have all made this possible. There are tremendous implications of obesity on individuals and society, including health systems and financial costs. Obesity alone accounts for nearly half of the $3.3 trillion spent annually on medical care for chronic conditions. Obesity prevalence continues to increase globally. According to the Centers for Disease Control and Prevention (CDC), the prevalence in the United States was 42.4% in 2017–2018 [1]. Worldwide, 39% of adults were overweight in 2016, and 13% were obese [2]. Notably, the worldwide obesity rate has tripled over the last 40 years. Obesity disproportionately affects different ethnic groups; nearly 50% of African American adults are obese.

2. Defining obesity as a chronic illness

Obesity is recognized as a complex, chronic and progressive disease by the World Health Organization (WHO) as well as multiple international medical and scientific societies, requiring lifelong treatment, monitoring, and control [3]. The CDC defines chronic disease as conditions lasting greater than one year that require ongoing medical attention or limit activities of daily living, or both. Obesity is associated with three of leading chronic diseases - heart disease, cancer, and type 2 diabetes. There are widespread consequences of obesity compared to normal or healthy weight for many serious health conditions, including all causes of death, hypertension, diabetes mellitus, coronary heart disease, stroke, and many cancers. Chronic diseases need to be treated and monitored for an individual's lifetime. While patients' chronic diseases may improve with management, relapse can and does happen.

Obesity affects not only individual physiology but also individual psychology. Pre-existing psychological conditions, as well as post-operative conditions that can be created or exacerbated after bariatric surgery, need to be understood, treated, and followed. Recognizing the interaction and impact of obesity on psychopathology, as well as how to identify and treat related psychological disorders, continues to be a work in progress for the obesity medicine field.

3. Obesity is a complex and multi-factorial disease

Obesity is a multifactorial, chronic, and progressive disease whose pathogenesis is tied to a strong genetic component as well as a multitude of hormonal, metabolic, psychological, cultural and behavioral factors.

Physiologically, the path to weight gain is defined by a positive energy balance which occurs when consumed calories (energy intake) exceeds used calories (energy expenditure) in the performance of basic biological functions, daily activities, and exercise [3]. A positive energy balance can be caused by overeating or by not getting enough physical activity. In addition, there are other conditions that affect energy balance and fat accumulation which do not involve excessive eating or sedentary behavior. These include:

Chronic sleep loss.

Chronic stress and psychological distress.

Consumption of foods that, independent of caloric content, cause metabolic/hormonal changes that can increase body fat – foods high in sugar or high fructose corn syrup, processed grains and meats, and fats.

Low intake of fat-fighting foods such as fruits, vegetables, legumes, nuts, seeds, quality protein.

Various medications – such as steroids and anti-depressants.

Various pollutants.

Weight gain is self-perpetuating, which is a reason why obesity is considered a progressive disease. Weight gain causes hormonal, metabolic and molecular changes that increase the potential for even greater fat accumulation. Obesity-associated biological changes reduce the body's ability to oxidize fat for energy, increase the conversion of glucose/carbohydrates to fat, and increase the body's capacity to store fat. This means that more calories consumed will end up being stored as fat. To worsen matters, obesity affects appetite and hunger regulators in a way that can decrease satiety, increasing portion size and eating frequency. Weight gain, therefore, changes the biology of the body in a manner that favors further weight gain and obesity [3].

Dieting to reduce caloric intake is a primary treatment for obesity, but it can also contribute to obesity progression. Dietary weight-loss causes biological responses that can persist long-term and end up contributing to weight regain. Weight loss can lead to reduced energy expenditure and calorie conservation if the body 'thinks' it is starving. A reduction in energy expenditure with dietary weight-loss requires that, to maintain weight-loss, an individual eat even fewer calories compared with someone of equal body size who has never dieted before. Eating less can be especially difficult with dieting, since there can be associated long-term changes in appetite regulation which increase hunger and food consumed. Such diet-induced changes favor a positive energy balance and weight regain. Since the conditions responsible reduced energy expenditure and increased appetite can persist long-term, an individual often will not only regain their lost weight, but even more [3].

Changes in fat metabolism are another biological response that occurs with dieting. Dietary weight-loss can lead to reduced oxidation of dietary fat by approximately 50 percent [4]. This includes reduced fat burning during low-grade activity such as walking, house chores, or working on a computer. This reduction in fat oxidation following a dietary weight-loss increases the amount of fat available for storage. In fact, dieting increases the capacity for fat depots to store even more fat than before a diet. These changes lead to a progressive increase in fat accumulation even if the individual is not overeating.

As a heritable trait, obesity is influenced by the interplay of genetics, epigenetics, metagenomics and the environment. Genetic predisposition to obesity is well studied and described [5, 6]. An example of this is a classic study of obesity within Danish adopted individuals, which demonstrated a high degree of correlation of body mass index (BMI) between adoptees and their biological parents, instead of their adoptive parents [5]. Another study by the same authors demonstrated that twins raised separately had similar BMI with each other, regardless of the environment in which they were raised [7]. Epigenetic changes may be involved as mediators of environmental influences and provide future opportunities for intervention [8].

Obesity can be associated with several endocrine alterations due to changes in the hypothalamic–pituitary hormones axis. These include hypothyroidism, Cushing's disease, hypogonadism, and growth hormone deficiency. Besides its role in energy storage, adipose tissue has several other important functions that can be mediated through hormones or substances synthesized and released by adipocytes, which include leptin and adiponectin. Additionally, obesity is also a common feature of polycystic ovarian syndrome with hyperinsulinemia being the primary etiological factor [9].

Metabolic syndrome is a condition characterized by a specific constellation of reversible major risk factors for cardiovascular disease and type 2 diabetes. The main diagnostic components are reduced HDL-cholesterol, raised triglycerides, blood pressure and fasting plasma glucose, all of which are related to weight gain, specifically intra-abdominal/ectopic fat accumulation and a large waist circumference. Metabolic syndrome is directly related to advancing age, affecting 30–40% of people by age 65. This seems to be driven mainly by progressive adult weight gain, and by a genetic or epigenetic predisposition to intra-abdominal/ectopic fat accumulation. Metabolic syndrome can also be associated with conversely, a lack of subcutaneous adipose tissue, low skeletal muscle mass and anti-retroviral drugs. Reducing weight even by only 5–10% substantially lowers all metabolic syndrome components, and the risk of type 2 diabetes and cardiovascular disease [10].

Culture also has a substantial association with BMI. This association is important for understanding the pattern of obesity across different cultures and countries. It is also important to recognize the importance of the association of culture and BMI in developing public health interventions to reduce obesity [11].

4. Psychology and behavior

Numerous studies support a strong link between obesity and mental health. This relationship is a two-way street; while mental health disorders increase the risk for obesity, having obesity also increases the risk of mental health disorders, especially in certain populations. Mental health disorders can increase the risk for obesity for various reasons. Medications used to treat psychiatric illnesses, such as anti-depressants, can themselves cause weight gain and insulin resistance. Additionally, mental illnesses are correlated with behaviors such as chronic sleep loss, poor eating behaviors, and sedentary behavior, which can contribute to obesity development.

Obesity increases the risk for depression. This is likely due to numerous complex factors, including poor self-esteem and depressed mood in response to weight bias and stigma, decreased activity and impaired mobility from joint and back pain associated with excess weight, and biological disruptions caused by adipocyte secretion of chemicals during obesity [12]. Obese patients overall have higher levels of stress, anxiety, depression, food craving, and emotional and behavioral disturbance [EBD] symptoms, with lower levels of self-esteem and quality of life compared with normal-weight individuals. Additionally, the severity of psychological disorders is directly related to the degree of obesity [12].

It is important that patients with mental health disorders are monitored for weight disorders, and that obese individuals are screened for mental health disorders. Treatment of obesity is associated with a significant improvement of anxiety, depression, and general psychopathology, and a similar pattern of reduction of binge eating symptomatology. Pre-treatment emotional eating severity has been found to be a significant outcome modifier, supporting the importance of a pre-treatment careful psychological assessment to supervise the post-surgical outcome [13].

Evaluation for underlying eating disorders such as food addiction and binge eating can be important assessment criteria for patients looking to undergo bariatric surgery, as well as for ongoing assessment afterwards. There are multiple surveys, questionnaires, and assessment tools that can be used to evaluate psychopathology before and after bariatric surgery. Examples include the Yale Food Addiction Scale (YFAS), Emotional Eating Scale, Beck Depression Inventory-Second Edition (BDI-II), Hospital Anxiety and Depression Scale, and the Short-Form Health Survey-36 (SF-36). These disorders share overlapping and non-overlapping features; the presence of both may represent a more severe obesity subgroup among treatment-seeking samples. Loss-of-control (LOC) eating, a key marker of binge eating, is one of the few consistent predictors of suboptimal weight outcomes post-bariatric surgery [14].

The presence of food addiction without binge eating has mixed results in terms of impact on weight loss after bariatric surgery. While some studies do not appear to show an impact [15], others show a correlation between higher number of food addiction symptoms and less weight loss [16]. Patients with emotional eating diagnosed pre-operatively, such as in response to anger/frustration, anxiety, or depression, are more likely to miss follow-up appointments and have poorer weight loss outcomes at 1-year post-op [16]. Evidence like this supports screening for these behaviors during the pre-surgical psychosocial evaluation, which would allow opportunities for psychotherapy and potential improvement in weight loss outcomes.

Psychiatric symptoms may not be related to weight loss outcomes [16]. Depressive disorders, as opposed to anxiety disorders, have been shown to decrease significantly after bariatric surgery. Importantly however, the presence of depressive disorders after bariatric surgery significantly predicts post-surgical outcomes and may signal a need for heightened clinical attention [17].

5. Behavior modification

Behavioral modification is an increasingly studied element of long-term obesity management. As a key component of obesity pathogenesis, behaviors before and after bariatric surgery are important but poorly documented or followed. Surgery, like medical therapy, is essentially an adjunct to what becomes a comprehensive, long-lasting management plan that addresses the multifactorial etiology of obesity.

Weekly self-weighing, eating cessation when feeling full, and not eating continuously during the day are three habits shown to improve post-operative weight loss by up to 14%, compared with individuals that do not engage in these behaviors [18]. Baseline cognitive restraint and strong adherence to the recommended postoperative diet are associated with an additional 4.5% weight loss after bariatric surgery [19]. Results like these suggest the importance of pre- and postoperative dietary counseling to improve postoperative outcomes. A significant minority of patients appear to experience suboptimal weight loss after bariatric surgery. The reasons for this are not well understood, but suboptimal weight loss is often attributed to preoperative psychosocial characteristics and/or eating behaviors, as well as poor adherence to a recommended postoperative diet.

Important components of long-term obesity management include assessing eating problems, weight control practices, and prior or current substance abuse such as the problematic use of alcohol, smoking, and illegal drugs. In addition to recognizing these detrimental factors, it is important to have a process in place to address problematic eating behaviors and eating patterns.

Preconditioning is an element of preparation for bariatric surgery that sets expectations, lays the groundwork for behavioral modification, and helps get candidates ready for a lifestyle change. It involves coursework and counseling by a multidisciplinary team on a one-on-one basis or in a group setting. This provides multiple perspectives and education by a dietitian, occupational and/or physical therapist, psychologist, and surgeon. Variations of preconditioning include the amount of coursework and didactics required, the need to pass exams, and objective clearance parameters by the multidisciplinary team. Nutritional education is a large part of preconditioning, since evaluating a candidate's relationship with food, triggers for eating, and implementation of management techniques for healthy eating is such a large part of long-term success with weight loss. Additionally, cognitive behavioral therapy courses can also be included. Intensive preconditioning in addition to close multidisciplinary follow-up postoperatively, has been shown to improve weight loss outcomes after bariatric surgery [20].

6. Predictors of weight loss

Predictors of weight loss outcomes after bariatric surgery fall can be categorized as: 1) presurgical factors, 2) postsurgical psychosocial variables (e.g., support group attendance), 3) postsurgical eating patterns, 4) postsurgical physical activity, and 5) follow-up at postsurgical clinic. There is varying evidence regarding these predictors and how well they correlate with success after bariatric surgery. However, the only factor which has been subjected to meta-analysis, and which shows a positive association with postoperative weight loss is preoperative weight loss. Other preoperatively identifiable factors associated with improved outcomes include Caucasian ethnicity or female gender [21], higher educational status, non-shiftwork working patterns, and divorced or single marital status [22].

Increased levels of preoperative physical activity and an absence of binge eating behavior also been linked with favorable results. Interestingly, increased age, smoking, a history of sexual abuse, or psychiatric illness have not been shown to have a significant impact. Conversely, diabetes mellitus seems to have a slight negative correlation with postoperative weight loss [22].

Other specific behavioral predictors associated with successful outcomes (e.g., ≥ 50% excess weight loss) are postoperative dietary adherence and support group attendance. Successful weight loss has been reported highest (92.6%) among patients reporting dietary adherence of >3 on a 9-point scale who graze no more than once-per-day. Post-operative patients with dietary adherence <3 but who graze daily or less have more than double the success rate of achieving >50% excess weight loss when their highest lifetime BMI is <53. Success rates also double for participants with low to moderate dietary adherence (3 or less) that attend support groups (either in-person or online) [23, 24]. While is unclear which specific components of these support groups are beneficial, or what constitutes optimal attendance frequency, it is possible that patients with low to moderate dietary adherence particularly benefit from the social support, accountability, and sharing of informational "tips" that promote adherence (i.e., cooking tips) [23, 24].

Alternatively, predictors of significant postoperative weight regain after bariatric surgery include indicators of baseline increased food urges, decreased well-being, and concerns over addictive behaviors. Postoperative self-monitoring behaviors are strongly associated with decreased weight regain. Data suggests that weight regain can be anticipated, in part, during the preoperative evaluation and potentially reduced with self-monitoring strategies after bariatric surgery [25]. Frequent self-weighing, at the very least, seems to be a good predictor of moderate weight loss, less weight regains, and avoidance of initial weight gain after surgery [26].

Given the chronic nature of obesity, patients after bariatric surgery should arguably be seeing a weight loss specialist for the remainder of their life. Especially after receiving a hypo absorptive operation, those patients should follow up with someone who is familiar with the specificities of their operation as well as pertinent side effects, nutritional deficiencies, etc. Long-term follow-up for patients after bariatric surgery is notoriously hard to achieve. There are multiple explanations of this, some of which are issues with the process, and others with the nature of the disease of chronic obesity. Weight loss programs sometimes do not set expectations for long term follow up in the beginning when patients start or reinforce this later. Resources can be present to get patients screened and set up for surgery but can be lacking post-operatively to keep patients engaged long-term. At some point, patients are often expected to continue follow up with their primary care physicians, who may or may not be familiar with the nuances of the type of bariatric procedure that the patient received or have the resources themselves to assist patients in staying on track or helping struggling patients with weight regain. Individual motivation can falter when it comes to follow up, or long-term adherence to nutritional and lifestyle changes that are important for maintaining weight loss.

Very few bariatric surgery studies report long-term results with sufficient patient follow-up to minimize biased results [27]. One study of a national bariatric surgery database in France showed that the percentage of patients with one or more visits to a surgeon dropped from 87.1% to 29.6% between year 1 and 6 after surgery. Predictors of poor 5-year follow-up include male sex, younger age, absence of type 2 diabetes and poor 1-year follow-up [28].

7. Other reasons for long-term follow-up

Many important long-term outcomes of bariatric surgery are still poorly understood, such as neurological and psychological complications, bone health, etc. Poor nutritional habits of obese people can result in baseline deficiency of several vitamins, minerals, and trace elements essential for body metabolism and normal physiological processes. Current bariatric surgical procedures such as sleeve gastrectomy, adjustable gastric banding, Roux-en-Y gastric bypass, and biliopancreatic diversion/duodenal switch can cause or exacerbate nutritional deficiencies and malnutrition, with different health implications unique to each surgery.

Purely restrictive operations such as adjustable gastric banding and sleeve gastrectomy affect the absorption of iron, selenium, and vitamin B12, while hypo absorptive operations such as gastric bypass and biliopancreatic diversion/duodenal switch have a more profound impact on the absorption of essential vitamins such as fat-soluble vitamins, minerals, and trace elements. Nutritional deficiencies in vitamins, minerals, and trace elements after bariatric surgery can result in clinical manifestations and diseases, such as anemia, ataxia, hair loss, and Wernicke encephalopathy [29].

Preoperative nutritional assessment and correction of vitamin and micronutrient deficiencies, as well as long-term postoperative nutritional follow-up, are important. Patient awareness, education and counseling start preoperatively, and continues after surgery. Dietetic counseling should continue frequently during the first year and be extended optionally afterwards, depending on individual and surgery specific factors. Vitamin supplementation should be discussed before surgery, with emphasis on specific needs required after surgery, and followed up on. Routine, relevant bloodwork should be obtained at appropriate intervals, with decrease in frequency as needed, but checks at least annually long term. Deviations from anticipated clinical course should prompt immediate reevaluation of nutritional levels. Planned and structured physical exercise should be systematically promoted to build and maintain muscle mass and improve bone health [30].

Weight loss programs utilizing bariatric surgery must implement robust, consistent, and evidence-based strategies to improve weight loss reduce weight regain. Long term follow up is an important factor in reinforcing behavioral modification necessary for long term weight loss, and monitoring for side effects possible after bariatric surgery. As adherence to long-term follow-up has been shown to decrease over time, it is important to identify measures that improve follow-up rates to get the maximum benefit from bariatric surgery, while minimizing long-term adverse effects and complications [31].

8. Conclusion

Obesity can be successfully treated, especially if approached in a comprehensive, multi-disciplinary, long-term fashion, as befits a complex and chronic disease. Important components of successful surgical management include careful patient selection, setting expectations, pre-conditioning, behavioral modification, and long-term postoperative follow-up. This requires screening and management of clinically impactful psychosocial diagnoses, comprehensive education and dietary counseling, access to support groups, and the resources to ensure follow-up postoperatively. Various bariatric surgical procedures, especially those with a hypo-absorptive component, are at risk for several nutrient deficiencies that need to be monitored long-term.

There remains a significant level of uncertainty regarding the best clinical practices for optimizing and maintaining weight loss after bariatric surgery. Standardization of bariatric surgical processes and guidelines by professional organizations such as the American Society for Metabolic and Bariatric surgeons (ASMBS) is an important start. However, more effort is needed to screen and improve psychological care, behavior management, and provide therapeutic patient education **after** surgery.

Understanding post-bariatric surgery outcome failure is important in addressing and helping the significant minority of patients (20–30%) who do not have expected weight loss, and subsequently regain weight previously lost. Screening for the multitude of risk factors related to bariatric surgery outcomes post-operatively can provide clinically relevant and useful information. For example, asking postsurgical patients to rate their level of adherence to dietary recommendations, and the frequency of grazing identifies high risk patients and the need for intervention. Additional measures based on patient's responses might include additional dietary assistance, referral for behavior therapy, and encouraged attendance at bariatric support groups. If return of appetite after surgery is an identified impediment with dietary adherence, evaluation for anti-obesity medications (AOMs) may be useful.

Additional investigation is needed into specific psychosocial, behavioral, and dietary adherence components that affect postsurgical weight loss outcome. Future research should determine how eating disorders such as food addiction affect long-term postoperative outcomes and mood stability, and examine which interventions are successful at improving problematic eating behaviors. It is also important to better understand patient motivational characteristics in relation to treatment compliance such as follow-up, support group participation and other aftercare recommendations. Results of this research will ultimately lead to better understanding of postsurgical outcome success and failure, and lead to better tailored yet standardized interventions accordingly.

Conflict of interest

The authors declare no conflict of interest.

Author details

Juaquito M. Jorge* and Frederick M. Tiesenga
Tiesenga Surgical Associates, S.C., Elmwood Park, Illinois, USA

*Address all correspondence to: jmjorge77@gmail.com

References

[1] Adult Obesity Facts. 2021. Available from: https://www.cdc.gov/obesity/data/adult.html

[2] Obesity and Overweight. 2021. Available from: https://www.who.int/news-room/fact-sheets/detail/obesity-and-overweight

[3] Disease of Obesity. 2022. Available from: https://asmbs.org/patients/disease-of-obesity

[4] Why Is Obesity a Disease? 2017. Available from: https://obesitymedicine.org/why-is-obesity-a-disease/

[5] Stunkard AJ, Sørensen TI, Hanis C, et al. An adoption study of human obesity. The New England Journal of Medicine. 1986;**314**(4):193-198. DOI: 10.1056/NEJM198601233140401

[6] Stunkard AJ. Genetic contributions to human obesity. Research Publications - Association for Research in Nervous and Mental Disease. 1991;**69**:205-218

[7] Stunkard AJ, Harris JR, Pedersen NL, McClearn GE. The body-mass index of twins who have been reared apart. The New England Journal of Medicine. 1990;**322**(21):1483-1487. DOI: 10.1056/NEJM199005243222102

[8] Thaker VV. Genetic and epigentic causes of obesity. Adolescent Medicine: State of the Art Reviews. 2017;**28**(2):379-405

[9] Sidhu S, Parikh T, Burman KD. Endocrine changes in obesity. [Updated 2017 Oct 12]. In: Feingold KR, Anawalt B, Boyce A, et al., editors. Endotext. South Dartmouth (MA): MDText.com, Inc.; 2000 Available from: https://www.ncbi.nlm.nih.gov/books/NBK279053/

[10] Han TS, Lean ME. A clinical perspective of obesity, metabolic syndrome and cardiovascular disease. JRSM Cardiovascular Disease. 2016;**5**:2048004016633371

[11] Masood M, Aggarwal A, Reidpath DD. Effect of national culture on BMI: A multilevel analysis of 53 countries. BMC Public Health. 2019;**19**:1212

[12] Abilés V, Rodríguez-Ruiz S, Abilés J, et al. Psychological characteristics of morbidly obese candidates for bariatric surgery. Obesity Surgery. 2010;**20**(2):161-167. DOI: 10.1007/s11695-008-9726-1

[13] Castellini G, Godini L, Amedei SG, Faravelli C, Lucchese M, Ricca V. Psychological effects and outcome predictors of three bariatric surgery interventions: A 1-year follow-up study. Eating and Weight Disorders. 2014;**19**(2):217-224. DOI: 10.1007/s40519-014-0123-6

[14] Ivezaj V, Wiedemann AA, Lawson JL, Grilo CM. Food addiction in sleeve gastrectomy patients with loss-of-control eating. Obesity Surgery. 2019;**29**(7):2071-2077. DOI: 10.1007/s11695-019-03805-8

[15] Koball AM, Clark MM, Collazo-Clavell M, et al. The relationship among food addiction, negative mood, and eating-disordered behaviors in patients seeking to have bariatric surgery. Surgery for Obesity and Related Diseases. 2016;**12**(1):165-170. DOI: 10.1016/j.soard.2015.04.009

[16] Miller-Matero LR, Bryce K, Saulino CK, Dykhuis KE, Genaw J, Carlin AM. Problematic eating Behaviors predict outcomes after bariatric surgery. Obesity Surgery. 2018;**28**(7):1910-1915. DOI: 10.1007/s11695-018-3124-0

[17] de Zwaan M, Enderle J, Wagner S, et al. Anxiety and depression in bariatric surgery patients: A prospective, follow-up study using structured clinical interviews. Journal of Affective Disorders. 2011;**133**(1-2):61-68. DOI: 10.1016/j.jad.2011.03.025

[18] Mitchell JE, Christian NJ, Flum DR, et al. Postoperative Behavioral variables and weight change 3 years after bariatric surgery. JAMA Surgery. 2016;**151**(8):752-757. DOI: 10.1001/jamasurg.2016.0395

[19] Sarwer DB, Wadden TA, Moore RH, et al. Preoperative eating behavior, postoperative dietary adherence, and weight loss after gastric bypass surgery. Surgery for Obesity and Related Diseases. 2008;**4**:4640-4646

[20] Matthew B, Flesher M, Sampath S, et al. The effect of intensive preconditioning and close follow-up on bariatric surgery outcomes: Does multidisciplinary care contribute to positive results whether a gastric bypass or sleeve gastrectomy is performed? BCMJ. Aug 2015;**57**(6):238-243

[21] Arterburn D, Livingston EH, Olsen MK, et al. Predictors of initial weight loss after gastric bypass surgery in twelve veterans affairs medical Centers. Obesity Research & Clinical Practice. 2013;**7**(5):e367-e376. DOI: 10.1016/j.orcp.2012.02.009

[22] Adams ST, Salhab M, Hussain ZI, Miller GV, Leveson SH. Roux-en-Y gastric bypass for morbid obesity: What are the preoperative predictors of weight loss? Postgraduate Medical Journal. 2013;**89**(1053):411-416. DOI: 10.1136/postgradmedj-2012-131310

[23] Robinson AH, Adler S, Stevens HB, Darcy AM, Morton JM, Safer DL. What variables are associated with successful weight loss outcomes for bariatric surgery after 1 year? Surgery for Obesity and Related Diseases. 2014;**10**(4):697-704. DOI: 10.1016/j.soard.2014.01.030

[24] Kaiser KA, Franks SF, Smith AB. Positive relationship between support group attendance and one-year postoperative weight loss in gastric banding. Surgery for Obesity and Related Diseases. 2011;**7**(1):89-93. DOI: 10.1016/j.soard.2010.07.013

[25] Odom J, Zalesin KC, Washington TL, et al. Behavioral predictors of weight regain after bariatric surgery. Obesity Surgery. 2010;**20**(3):349-356. DOI: 10.1007/s11695-009-9895-6

[26] Vanwormer JJ, French SA, Pereira MA, Welsh EM. The impact of regular self-weighing on weight management: A systematic literature review. International Journal of Behavioral Nutrition and Physical Activity. 2008;**5**:54. DOI: 10.1186/1479-5868-5-54

[27] Puzziferri N, Roshek TB 3rd, Mayo HG, Gallagher R, Belle SH, Livingston EH. Long-term follow-up after bariatric surgery: A systematic review. Journal of the American Medical Association. 2014;**312**(9):934-942. DOI: 10.1001/jama.2014.10706

[28] Thereaux J, Lesuffleur T, Païta M, Czernichow S, Basdevant A, Msika S, et al. Long-term follow-up after bariatric surgery in a national cohort. British Journal of Surgery. 2017;**104**(10):1362-1371. DOI: 10.1002/bjs.10557

[29] Gasmi A, Bjørklund G, Mujawdiya PK, et al. Micronutrients deficiences in patients after bariatric surgery. European Journal of Nutrition. 2022;**61**(1):55-67. DOI: 10.1007/s00394-021-02619-8

[30] Thibault R, Huber O, Azagury DE, Pichard C. Twelve key nutritional issues

in bariatric surgery. Clinical Nutrition. 2016;**35**(1):12-17. DOI: 10.1016/j.clnu. 2015.02.012

[31] Montastier E, du Rieu Maeld C, Tuyeras G, Ritz P. Long-term nutritional follow-up post bariatric surgery. Current Opinion in Clinical Nutrition and Metabolic Care. 2018;**21**(5):388-393. DOI: 10.1097/MCO.0000000000000490

Chapter 6

Current and Potential Applications of Artificial Intelligence in Metabolic Bariatric Surgery

Athanasios G. Pantelis

Abstract

Artificial intelligence (AI) is an umbrella term, which refers to different methods that simulate the process of human learning. As is the case with medicine in general, the field of bariatric metabolic surgery has lately been overwhelmed by evidence relevant to the applications of AI in numerous aspects of its clinical practice, including prediction of complications, effectiveness for weight loss and remission of associated medical problems, improvement of quality of life, intraoperative features, and cost-effectiveness. Current studies are highly heterogeneous regarding their datasets, as well as their metrics and benchmarking, which has a direct impact on the quality of research. For the non-familiar clinician, AI should be deemed as a novel statistical tool, which, in contradistinction to traditional statistics, draws their source data from real-world databases and registries rather than idealized cohorts of patients and is capable of managing vast amounts of data. This way, AI is supposed to support decision-making rather than substitute critical thinking or surgical skill development. As with any novelty, the clinical usefulness of AI remains to be proven and validated against established methods.

Keywords: artificial intelligence, machine learning, deep learning, data mining, decision trees, bariatric surgery, metabolic surgery, obesity, diabetes mellitus, obesity-related health problems, surgical safety, effectiveness, quality of life

1. Introduction

Artificial intelligence (AI) is an umbrella term that incorporates concepts such as supervised and unsupervised machine learning (ML), deep learning (DL), and reinforcement learning [1]. In essence, AI is the simulation of human learning by a machine (computer). Learning, in turn, is the procedure of acquiring information (input), which, after retention and processing, may lead to adjustment of behavior under given temporospatial circumstances or optimization of the chances of achieving specific goals (output). Each type of AI differs from the others in the extent of intervention by the operator, i.e., the degree of autonomy of the machine.

AI subtypes have certain integral components: an algorithm, specific datasets (training, validation, test), input (predictors), and output (outcomes), as well as performance indices of the algorithm for each dataset (sensitivity, specificity, F1 score, area under the receiver operator curve—AUROC, area under the precision-recall curve—AUPRC, and so on). Depending on the degree of autonomy of the AI algorithm, the operator (human researcher, data scientist) has variable knowledge of and interference to the aforementioned components. For instance, in *supervised ML,* the training data are labeled, and the possible outcomes are known *a priori*. This type of AI is used in cases of classification (in the case of categorical outcomes—i.e., disease or no disease, TNM staging for neoplasia, Clavien-Dindo staging for postoperative complications, etc.) or regression (in the case of numerical outcomes—i.e. weight, height, body mass index, etc.). Examples of supervised ML algorithms are decision trees (DT), random forest (RF), k-nearest neighbors (knn), linear and logistic regression (LR), support vector machines (SVMs), etc. On the other hand, in *unsupervised ML*, outcomes are unknown; therefore, they are subject to discovery with the aid of the AI algorithm itself. Unsupervised ML problems are divided into clustering (inherent grouping of data) and association (rules that define the relationship between predictors and outcomes). Besides, *reinforcement learning* is based on continuous training of the algorithm with the method of "trial-and-error" and is implemented in the case of highly chaotic systems such as cost analysis, with Markov models being typical examples [2].

Deep learning (DL) is the most autonomous subtype of AI. DL utilizes large amounts of real-world data (big data) and is structured on the basis of neural networks of three or more layers (input layer, output layer, one or more hidden intermediate layers). The layered architecture of DL algorithms resembles that of neurons in the central nervous system, hence the characterization "neural (or neuronal) networks." Characteristic examples are artificial neural networks (ANN), convolutional neural networks (CNNs), long-short term memory networks (LSTMNs), recurrent neural networks (RNNs), multilayer perceptrons (MLPs), etc. [2]. **Figure 1** is a

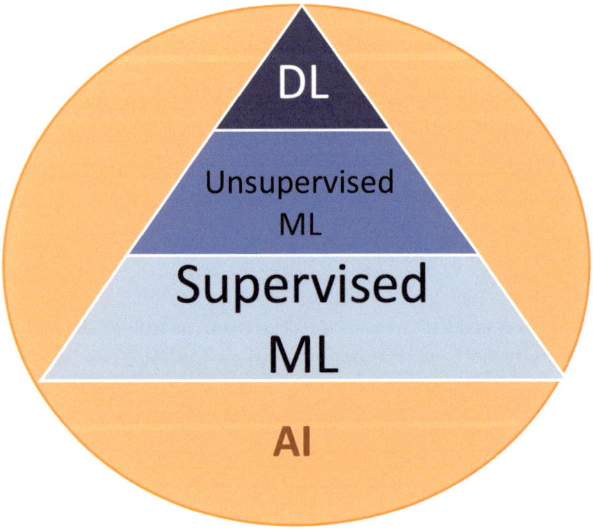

Figure 1.
Schematic representation of the hierarchy of artificial intelligence algorithms. The more one moves to the top of the pyramid, the more autonomous the algorithm becomes and the less intervention is exerted by the researcher. AI — artificial intelligence, ML — machine learning, DL — deep learning.

schematic representation of the different subtypes of AI, with the degree of autonomy of each one.

Recently there has been documented an exponential increase of literature investigating the application of various AI algorithms in healthcare [3]. It is within this context that our team recently attempted to trace the applications of artificial intelligence and machine learning in bariatric metabolic surgery (BMS) [4]. Based upon this study, this chapter is organized in seven sections, in concordance with the respective disciplines of BMS for which there have been relevant publications concerning applications of AI. The last two sections are devoted to the future perspectives of AI in BMS, as well as the methodological limitations and ethical barriers that should be considered when applying AI in BMS, in analogy to every biomedical scientific field.

2. AI applications in basic science relevant to bariatric metabolic surgery

Basic science and research are the cornerstones of evolution in medicine. Popular basic science applications on which AI may be applied include but are not limited to genome-wide sequencing (WGS), whole slide imaging (WSI), and all the omics (genomics, transcriptomics, proteomics, metabolomics, but also radiomics and multi-omics). Regarding the discipline of BMS in particular, metabolomics is a field of increased interest and intensive research, for the purpose of characterizing the metabolic milieu of patients living with obesity as well as for studying the long-term postoperative interactions between BMS and the metabolism [5–7].

In one of the first attempts to implement AI methods in BMS, Cortón et al. studied the gene expression profile in omental adipose tissue procured by women who were submitted to bariatric surgery and simultaneously suffered from polycystic ovarian syndrome (PCOS) [8]. More specifically, the researchers implemented data mining, a method that combines traditional statistics, machine learning and database systems, and retrieved abnormal expression of genes that participate in insulin and Wnt signaling, oxidative stress, inflammation, immune function, and lipid metabolism. Additionally, they conducted hierarchical clustering, a type of unsupervised ML, in order to retrieve co-expressed genes in female patients with PCOS and consequently detect specific patterns of gene expression.

More recently, Chaim et al. calculated beta cell function through assessment of NO production by means of electro-sensor complex (ESC) data and statistical network, a set of DL algorithms [9]. Subjects consisted of patients living with obesity who were candidates for MBS. In another study, Macartney-Coxson et al. used genome-wide DNA methylation data and compared traditional statistics with combinatorial algorithms in the identification of methylation loci [10]. Study samples included subcutaneous and omental adipose tissue that had been harvested from obese individuals, before and after BMS. Besides, Candi et al. performed a metabolomics analysis of visceral adipose tissue harvested from individuals who had undergone bariatric surgery and identified three kinds of metabolotypes: healthy controls (normal weight), healthy obese, and pathological obese [11]. Consequently, they implemented RF analysis, an unbiased supervised classification technique, in order to differentiate among the three groups, but also retrieve the most important predictive metabolites for each category, with lipids playing a cardinal role with this respect. In another metabolomics-oriented study, Narath et al. used an untargeted approach that yielded 177 features [12]. Consequently, they processed the data with RF in order to detect short- and long-term metabolic changes following Roux-en-Y gastric bypass (RYGB).

The most important finding was that short-term changes in metabolites (1–3 weeks postoperatively) do not necessarily match long-term effects (up to 1 year).

Future research should focus on reconciling metabolic surgery, metabolomics, and deep learning. So far, application of DL in metabolomics has manifested several methodological limitations, including high computational cost, lack of external validation, non-calculation of isotopic peaks during sample analysis with spectroscopy, overfitting secondary to low sample size, reduced predictive ability upon application to asymmetrical datasets, poor applicability of outcomes from experimental animal models to human metabolomics, etc. [13]. On the other hand, the exponentially increasing numbers of patients who undergo BMS offer an excellent substrate for obtaining biological fluids (whole blood, plasma, serum, feces, urine) and tissues (gastric, adipose, liver) for further metabolomic analysis. The implementation of ML, and most importantly DL, could potentially assist in unraveling the roles of the myriads of metabolites through untargeted metabolomic analyses, distinguish between causes and effects, and gain clinical usefulness both for prediction and diagnosis. With this regard, one may distinguish the emerging role of data analysists as key members of the multidisciplinary BMS team.

3. AI and surgical safety: predicting and preventing complications following bariatric metabolic surgery

Bariatric operations have a favorable safety profile, with an overall morbidity less than 5% and mortality less than 0.5%, as it has been documented over time by different investigators, based on data from large databases and comprehensive meta-analyses [14–20]. Most importantly, this holds true even for special populations, such as patients suffering from diabetes [21] or at the extremes of age [22, 23]. Even during the COVID-19 pandemic, not only has bariatric surgery proven its endurable safety, but it may also have a protective effect for one of the most vulnerable population groups against the adverse sequelae of SARS-CoV-2 [24, 25], as shown in a series of publications by the GENEVA collaborative group regarding 7704 patients from 42 countries [26–30]. Due to the fact that complications and deaths following BMS are rare events, their evaluation from a statistical perspective is challenging. Thanks to artificial intelligence algorithms, it is now possible to incorporate and analyze data from big databases and cohorts of patients, with the advantage of yielding reliable results from imbalanced datasets, as well as having access to real-word conditions rather than idealized simulations, as is the case with randomized controlled trials. Besides, the concept of implementing AI algorithms in order to quantify and predict postoperative outcomes, with the intention to enhance clinical practice and improve decision-making, is gaining popularity within surgical literature [31–33].

Cao et al. pioneered research in prediction of serious complications after BMS by implementing machine learning [34], as well as deep learning methods [35], in a Scandinavian bariatric database (SOReg) comprising more than 40,000 bariatric patients. In their extensive analyses, they compared multiple machine and deep learning algorithms (as well as combinations of algorithms, *aka* ensembles), respectively, and they found that the latter had better predictive accuracy, along with the fact that ensemble algorithms had better performance than baseline ones. Additionally, in order to overcome the obstacle of imbalanced data secondary to the low occurrence of complications, they applied the synthetic minority oversampling technique (SMOTE). SMOTE is a method of artificially augmenting underrepresented groups (such as patients with postoperative complications) and thus yield data eligible for classification. In a similar manner, Razzaghi et al. developed predictive models for bariatric surgery risks with imbalanced data by applying SMOTE on different classification algorithms, such as RF, bagging, and AdaBoost [36]. As a source of data, they utilized the Premier Healthcare Database, which gathers data from more than 700 hospitals across the United States. Again, their work showcased that ensemble classification was superior to isolated ML algorithms. Charles-Nelson followed a different strategy: in order to document the 30-day readmission rate, which is a reflection of short- and intermediate-term complications, they applied Formal Concept Analysis (FCA), a data mining technique, in a cohort of 196,323 bariatric patients according to the main principal diagnoses code at readmission [37]. Their most important finding was heterogeneity of severity of complications across different bariatric procedures.

There are two studies regarding prediction of complications after specific operations. Wise et al. applied a DL algorithm (ANN) on a cohort of 101,721 patients from the Metabolic and Bariatric Surgery Accreditation and Quality Improvement Program (MBSAQIP) who had undergone laparoscopic sleeve gastrectomy (LSG), in order to predict 30-day postoperative morbidity [38]. As compared with logistic regression, the ANN algorithm was more accurate in predicting postoperative complications, based upon easily obtainable demographic and clinical factors. Similarly, Sheikhtaheri et al. applied Clinical Decision Support System (CDSS) to predict morbidity after one-anastomosis gastric bypass (OAGB) across five hospitals over a 4-year period [39]. The predictive performance of the model at the 10-day, 1-month, and 3-months intervals was favorable.

Regarding specific complications, Dang et al. developed the BariClot tool, a forward regression predictive model, in order to stratify individuals undergoing BMS according to their 30-day risk for venous thromboembolic (VTE) events [40]. Their data were retrieved from the MBSAQIP and included patients who had undergone either RYGB or LSG. As compared with established predictive tools for VTE, such as the Michigan Bariatric Surgery Collaborative or the Caprini score, BariClot demonstrated enhanced predictive accuracy, as documented by the relevant AUROCs (0.5817 vs. 0.5533 vs. 0.6023, respectively). Moreover, Nudel et al. developed and validated three different machine/deep learning models (ANN, X-Gradient Boosting, logistic regression) in order to predict not only VTE, but also leaks after BMS, again based on a MBSAQIP cohort of 436,807 patients [41]. AI models outperformed traditional LR in detecting both leak and VTE in a statistically significant manner.

Finally, AI has also been implemented for predicting long-term morbidity after BMS, including the development of gallbladder disease and formation of gallstones [42], nutritional deficiencies [43], nonalcoholic fatty liver disease (NAFLD) [44], and fractures [45]. The implemented AI algorithms were ANN [42], SVM [44], and Bayesian networks [43, 45].

4. AI as a tool for predicting effectiveness of bariatric surgery

Undoubtedly, the main and utmost priority of any bariatric operation is weight loss. It has been long established that any bariatric intervention is more effective and durable in maintaining weight loss than optimal conservative treatment and lifestyle modifications [46–53]. Data that support this statement stem from both observational and randomized controlled studies. Although the latter are prospective in nature and thus can establish causality, they may be accompanied by publication bias. On the contrary, observational studies contain raw data as they are collected according to healthcare providers' registrations and patient testimonials. As such, they can serve as an invaluable source of prediction, provided they undergo appropriate analysis with AI tools. Nevertheless, despite the accumulated experience and evidence with bariatric surgery and its effectiveness, to date there is no accurate tool for weight loss prediction, and most clinical models tend to overestimate the bariatric outcome of the most commonly performed procedures [54].

In one of the first relevant attempts, Lee et al. developed a predictive model back in 2007 with the use of a data mining technology through LR and ANN [55]. They found that ANN yields a better predictive accuracy for weight reduction at 2 years as compared with traditional methods, with the best predictors of successful weight loss being OAGB (vs. LAGB), high preoperative triglyceride level, and low glycated hemoglobin (HbA1c) level. Similarly, Giraud-Carrier et al. developed a predictive model with the use of a data-mining-based software available online [56]. The data mining process included problem formulation (prediction of the type of bariatric procedure and quality of its outcome); domain and data understanding (71,849 patients with >350,000 visits across 125 centers); data preparation and preprocessing (aka determination of input or predictors, i.e., physician ID, gender, age, ethnicity, employment status, smoking behavior, state of origin, BMI prior to surgery, surgery performed, and BMI at 12 months postoperatively); model building (multinomial logistic regression and decision tree C4.5); prediction of surgical procedure; prediction of success (classification into poor, fair, good, very good, and excellent if BMI reduction at 12 months was ≤5, 5–10, 10–15, 15–20, and >20, respectively). Although these studies were performed at an era when experience on bariatric surgery was more limited, the armamentarium of procedures was significantly different, benchmarking was inadequate, and definition of weight loss was not according to current standards (%TWL or %EBMIL or %EBMIL), the study designs showed a dynamic potential. More recent attempts have implemented different methodology (i.e., a rule-based semantic approach, [57]) or different input data (i.e., preoperative patient liking for sweet beverages, [58]) in order to predict bariatric surgery outcomes in general.

Other studies have focused on specific bariatric operations. For instance, Piaggi et al. found that ANN models could successfully predict weight loss in women treated with laparoscopic adjustable gastric banding (LAGB), although this method tends to be abandoned nowadays [59]. On the other hand, Celik et al. in a very recent study applied neural network Bayesian regularization, a DL algorithm, in patients who had undergone LSG and predicted excess and total weight loss (%EWL and %TWL, respectively) based on gastric remnant volumes (antrum and body were deemed as different compartments) [60]. Regarding RYGB, Wise ES *et al.* implemented an ANN model to predict excess weight loss by means of % reduction in BMI loss (%EBMIL) at 3 months and 1 year postoperatively [61]. On a more advanced level, Choudhury et al. implemented a Markov model so as to predict which modality of weight loss was more effective for patients with end-stage renal disease awaiting renal transplant [62]. Not surprisingly, RYGB was found to be more effective than aggressive diet and exercise with this regard.

5. AI as a tool for diagnosing and predicting resolution of obesity-associated medical problems after bariatric metabolic surgery

Apart from weight loss, MBS is associated with the alleviation of the long-term effects of associated medical problems (or comorbidity, as they were collectively referred to until recently), namely type 2 diabetes mellitus (T2DM), hypertension (HTN), nonalcoholic fatty liver disease (NAFLD), and nonalcoholic steatohepatitis (NASH), obstructive sleep apnea (OSA), dyslipidemia, end-stage renal disease (ESRD), depression, etc. Most importantly, some of these health problems have been recognized as dedicated indications for MBS, irrespective of BMI [63]. The rationale of this is supported by high-quality evidence on the superiority of surgical management vs. intensive medical therapy [64, 65]. Regarding T2DM in particular, the evidence is solid and stems from cohorts with long-term perspective surveillance [66–69], to the point that they have substantially contributed to the establishment of the concept of metabolic surgery in clinical practice [70, 71].

The advent of AI has introduced novel methods of predicting long-term remission of obesity-associated medical problems based on real-world data. In a recent comprehensive relevant study, Cao et al. compared three different AI models (Gaussian Bayesian Network – GBN, CNN, and traditional linear regression) in predicting 5-year remission of T2DM, dyslipidemia, HTN, OSA, and depression from data extracted from the large SOReg database concerning 6542 patients [72]. Among the examined algorithms, GBN showed excellent performance in predicting long-term remission of T2DM (AUC 0.942) and dyslipidemia (AUC 0.917), good performance for HTN (AUC 0.891) and OSA (AUC 0.843), and fair performance in predicting depression (AUC 0.750). On the other hand, van Loon et al. devised the Metabolic Health Index (MHI) to objectively quantify metabolic health, in analogy to BMI as an index for quantifying weight, and consequently developed an ordinal logistic regression model in order to quantify severity of comorbidity in a 6-grade scale [73]. As a scaffold, they used 4778 data records from 1595 patients and high-yield predictors included age, estimated glomerular filtration rate (eGFR), HbA1c, triglycerides, and potassium.

Regarding specific conditions, T2DM has been the most studied obesity-associated health problem with regard to AI algorithms so far. Lee et al. ran a series of multi-centric studies with the aim to investigate the effectiveness of BMS in T2DM resolution, as well as to predict short- and long-term T2DM remission after BMS [74–76]. Their analysis was performed by means of back propagation neural networks (BPN), a type of ANN, and important predictors of T2DM remission included younger patient age, shorter T2DM duration, higher weight, wider waist, higher C-peptide levels, and bypass operation (vs. restrictive one). A few years later, another group investigated the role of the advanced-Diabetes Remission (ad-DiaRem) score in improving the prediction of T2DM remission following RYGB [77, 78]. DiaRem is a valid prediction score for T2DM remission that relies on variables such as age, HbA1c, treatment with insulin, treatment with oral hypoglycemics other than metformin and classifies patients into five subgroups according to their probability of remission [79–81]. Ad-DiaRem has two additional parameters (diabetes duration and number of glucose-lowering agents). The group of Aron-Wisnewsky, Debédat et al. analyzed Ad-DiaRem with the use of machine learning and devised a 1-year algorithm with enhanced predictive accuracy as compared with the original score, which yielded a corrected classification for 8% of those misclassified with DiaRem [77]. The same team used

ML methods to extend the predictive accuracy to 5 years post-RYGB, with the correct re-classification rate reaching 33% [78]. Consequently, AI can be implemented not only as a novel method, but also in order to improve established clinical tools.

At a more advanced level, Aminian et al. utilized ML in order to predict long-term end-organ complications owing to T2DM (in particular all cause-mortality, coronary artery events, heart failure, and nephropathy) in patients who did or did not undergo metabolic surgery [82]. A total of 2287 T2DM patients who had undergone metabolic operations were matched with 11,435 non-surgical diabetic patients. Analysis was performed by means of multivariable regression and random forest and data were uploaded by patients through user-friendly web-based and smartphone applications in an Individualized Diabetes Complications (IDC) risk score environment for clinical use. This is one of the most useful applications of ML in clinical practice so far. In another sophisticated study, Pedersen et al. combined clinical data (treatment with insulin, use of insulin-sensitizing agents, baseline HbA1c levels, and baseline serum insulin levels) with eight single-nucleotide polymorphisms (SNPs) and processed the data with ANN [83]. The addition of the SNPs significantly improved the predictive ability of the algorithm.

Nonalcoholic fatty liver disease (NAFLD)/nonalcoholic steatohepatitis (NASH) constitutes another entity of particular interest in the context of obesity. NAFLD/NASH represents the most common chronic liver disease worldwide nowadays, for the treatment of which BMS seems to play a pivotal role as it seems to offer sustainable resolution [84–86]. Back in 2013, Sowa et al. examined several ML algorithms (among which LR, knn, SVM, decision trees, RF) to determine noninvasive assessment of fibrosis in NAFLD based on serum parameters (transaminases, hyaluronic acid, and cell death markers) and compared their combined effect with the gold standard of liver biopsy, which was performed intraoperatively during BMS [87]. The combination of these parameters with RF had a better diagnostic accuracy than each single parameter. More recently, Uehara et al. constructed a noninvasive algorithm for predicting NASH in a Japanese population of patients living with morbid obesity [88]. The most important predictors (alanine aminotransferase—ALT, C-reactive protein—CRP, homeostasis model assessment insulin resistance—HOMA-IR, and albumin) were selected by means of rule extraction technology.

6. AI as a means of improving quality of life assessment following bariatric metabolic surgery

Quality of life (QoL) after BMS is a parameter with increasing interest in literature because it is perhaps more patient-related and less of a technicality, as compared with safety, effectiveness, and resolution of associated health problems. There are several scores for evaluating QoL after BMS and their applicability has been implemented after various procedures [89–92]. In the realm of AI, the group of Cao et al. has conducted two studies based on the SOReg with the use of CNN, Gaussian Bayesian Network (BN), and LR for predicting 5-year health-related QoL after BMS [72, 93]. GBN showed better predictive accuracy as compared with the other methods. In another publication, BN was implemented for a network meta-analysis of studies referring to QoL after BMS [94]. The analysis involved 26,629 patients in total and 11 different procedures.

7. AI for evaluating intraoperative aspects of bariatric metabolic surgery

One of the advantages of laparoscopic surgery (and video-assisted surgery in general) is the continuous recording of the procedure. In the digital era, these recordings can be transformed into captions, which subsequently may be stored, transferred, processed, etc. Another usage that has recently been highlighted is technical skill assessment. In comparison to crude measures of surgical performance, such as operative time, postoperative outcomes, and complications, video-assisted operative evaluation offers better opportunities for constructive feedback and progressive improvement of technique. The rating may be performed by human peers and supervisors, but lately ML has shown promising results in objective assessment of surgical skills [95].

In the field of BMS specifically, Twinanda et al. have pioneered AI techniques in laparoscopic videos with two discrete applications: retrieval of a specific fraction of the video (i.e., suturing of an anastomosis) and prediction of remaining time. In the former example, the researchers used Fisher kernel encoding, a precursor of deep learning techniques for managing large-scale object categorization, and applied it on 49 bypass and seven LSG videos [96]. In the latter case, remaining operative time in 170 RYGB videos was predicted by RSDNet, a DL-based algorithm that depends only on visual data for training rather than manual annotations [97]. Other pioneers in computer vision analysis of operative steps are Hashimoto et al., who implemented DNN to analyze LSG videos [98]. In this case, laparoscopic videos were segmented into seven steps: port placement, liver retraction, liver biopsy, gastrocolic ligament dissection, stapling of the stomach along the greater curvature, bagging specimen, and final inspection of the staple line. AI could extract quantitative data from video with an accuracy of >85%, a feature that allows quantification of operative capacity and objective evaluation for the purposes of both training and self-development. Similarly, Derathé et al. utilized annotated spatial and procedural data and processed them with SVM in order to predict surgical exposure [99].

In a totally different approach, Heremans et al. implemented ANN-based automated detection of food intake after neuromodulation by analyzing heart rate variability in electrocardiograms [100]. This is another example of intraoperative application of AI in a different kind of surgery for weight loss (neuromodulation).

8. Cost analysis of bariatric metabolic surgery with the use of AI

We are living in an era that cost-effectiveness is paramount in medicine for every intervention, either conservative or surgical. It has been estimated that the cost of BMS is approximately 14,000 euros and 3600 euros annually ever after. In comparison, the cost for the non-surgical treatment of T2DM is about 12,200 euros per annum [101].

Cost analyses are considered dynamic systems that are affected by various, often non-predicable parameters. Many cost analyses studies are based on Markov models. Markov models are stochastic models designed for systems that change over time (i.e., dynamic ones) and change their parameters randomly. Using decision analysis with the implementation of a Markov process, Borisenko et al. calculated that the annual savings for a cohort of bariatric patients from the SOReg was 66 million euros, whereas over a lifetime bariatric surgery produced savings of 9332 euros [102, 103].

Similarly, Faria et al. compared different bariatric interventions and calculated that RYGB saves an average of 13,244 euros per patient as compared with best medical management [104].

9. AI: hope or hype? methodological, ethical, medicolegal issues, and patient perspectives

AI is a relatively novel clinical tool, as such the healthcare provider should be cautious before adopting its methods and incorporating them into clinical routine. The following limitations are uniform across medicine, not BMS alone, and prompt the implementation of a solid frame in the context of which AI may yield its most beneficial aspects in clinical practice. Extensive analysis of AI limitations is beyond the scope of this chapter; therefore, we will attempt to outline the most important aspects of them.

One of the advantages of AI is the management of large amounts of data, but at the same time this is a prerequisite to obtain reliable outcomes. As such, data quantity is one issue. Data quality is another, and this can be achieved only when source data (i.e., registries or electronic health records—EHRs) are comprehensive and inclusive. In other words, all patients should have access to health services irrespective of socioeconomic status, and health services on their part should promote continuity of care instead of segmentation. The third important component is model interpretation, especially when it comes to deep learning, given that sometimes the relations between inputs (predictors) and outcomes are not obvious. Next, model generalizability and interoperability are paramount for implementing AI algorithms across different health systems and contexts, and these can be ensured only when the three former methodological requirements are met. Finally, AI researchers must ensure model security, i.e., avoid "contamination" of data. This is a potential issue even after meticulous training of data [105]. To address these potential sources of bias, several strategies have been proposed. Among them, oversampling minority groups in training datasets, creating flags for certain high-risk groups, and formulating baseline predictions at presentation of illness (i.e., in the case of BMS, before surgery) are the most feasible ones [106].

The usage of AI as a decision-making tool may also have medicolegal sequelae. In this case, one should take into consideration all the parameters, i.e., agreement between AI recommendation and standard of care, accuracy of AI prediction, physician action (acceptance or rejection of the AI decision), and patient outcome. Different combinations may lead to different legal outcomes, i.e., no injury of the patient and no liability of the surgeon, injury but no liability, or both injury and liability [107]. Consequently, on the one hand, healthcare providers should know how to interpret AI algorithm outcomes and recruit their clinical judgment above all; on the other hand, they should have an active role in shaping their liability issue through their professional societies and legislation-forming organizations.

Is the role of the surgeon threatened by the advent of AI? Are surgeons transforming from leaders to simple operators of what a machine has decided for a patient? Definitely not. AI should be deemed as a tool that is intended to assist surgeons in their daily workflow and ease their work with the intent to help them focus on what is important, i.e., physician-patient relationship. Additionally, AI offers a real opportunity for individualized interventions and precision medicine, not only at the time of operations, must (even most importantly) during the postoperative period and follow-up.

What impact does AI make on patients themselves? According to a recently published survey, it depends on the context. Fifty-five percent of participants were very or somewhat comfortable with AI making chest X-ray diagnosis, but the respective percentage for making cancer diagnosis dropped to 31.2% [108]. Consequently, the role of the surgeon remains central to continuum of healthcare provision, while discussing all diagnostic and therapeutic options with the patient is indispensable.

As it has been stressed out by Bellini et al., AI has contributed to substantial progress in decision-making, quality of care, and precision medicine, but several legal and ethical issues need to be addressed before its widespread application in clinical practice [109].

10. Conclusions

AI is gaining more and more ground to clinical practice, as it has been documented not only by our research [4], but also that of other investigators within the same context [109]. The clinician is not required to understand how AI algorithms work but should be cautious when interpreting AI-based outcomes and decision by evaluating its source data and metrics. For reasons of simplicity, AI should be considered a novel statistical tool with the advantage of yielding data from large, real-world registries of patients rather than restricted cohorts as the ones used in the context of randomized trials. Given the specialized nature of processing these data, specialists such as data scientists could assume new roles in the multidisciplinary team of managing bariatric patients.

Conflict of interest

The author declares no conflict of interest.

Author details

Athanasios G. Pantelis
4th Department of Surgery, Bariatric Metabolic Surgery Unit, Evaggelismos General Hospital of Athens, Athens, Greece

*Address all correspondence to: ath.pantelis@gmail.com

References

[1] Loftus TJ, Tighe PJ, Filiberto AC, et al. Artificial Intelligence and Surgical Decision-making. JAMA Surgery. 2020;**155**(2):148-158. DOI: 10.1001/jamasurg.2019.4917

[2] AI with Python Tutorial. 2016. Available from: https://www.tutorialspoint.com/artificial_intelligence_with_python/ index.htm

[3] Yu KH, Beam AL, Kohane IS. Artificial intelligence in healthcare. Nature Biomedical Engineering. 2018;**2**(10):719-731. Available from: https://pubmed.ncbi.nlm.nih.gov/31015651/

[4] Pantelis AG, Stravodimos GK, Lapatsanis DP. A scoping review of artificial intelligence and machine learning in bariatric and metabolic surgery: Current status and future perspectives. Obesity Surgery. 2021;**31**(10):4555-4563. Available from: https://pubmed.ncbi.nlm.nih.gov/34264433/

[5] Samczuk P, Ciborowski M, Kretowski A. Application of metabolomics to study effects of bariatric surgery. Journal of Diabetes Research. 2018;**2018**:13. Article ID 6270875. https://doi.org/10.1155/2018/6270875

[6] Ha J, Jang M, Kwon YK, Park YS, Park DJ, Lee JH, et al. Metabolomic profiles predict diabetes remission after bariatric surgery. Journal of Clinical Medicine. 2020;**9**(12):1-12. Available from: https://pubmed.ncbi.nlm.nih.gov/33271740/

[7] Vaz M, Pereira SS, Monteiro MP. Metabolomic signatures after bariatric surgery – a systematic review.Reviews in Endocrine and Metabolic Disorders. 2022;**23**:503-519. https://doi.org/10.1007/s11154-021-09695-5

[8] Cortón M, Botella-Carretero JI, Benguría A, Villuendas G, Zaballos A, San Millán JL, et al. Differential gene expression profile in omental adipose tissue in women with polycystic ovary syndrome. The Journal of Clinical Endocrinology and Metabolism. 2007;**92**(1):328-337. Available from: https://pubmed.ncbi.nlm.nih.gov/17062763/

[9] Chaim EA, Gobato RC. New approach to beta cell function screening by nitric oxide assessment of obese individuals at the population level. International Journal of General Medicine. 2012;**5**: 449-454. Available from: https://pubmed.ncbi.nlm.nih.gov/22675263/

[10] Macartney-Coxson D, Benton MC, Blick R, Stubbs RS, Hagan RD, Langston MA. Genome-wide DNA methylation analysis reveals loci that distinguish different types of adipose tissue in obese individuals. Clinical Epigenetics. 2017;**9**(1):48. PMCID: PMC5415776. DOI: 10.1186/s13148-017-0344-4. Available from: https://pubmed.ncbi.nlm.nih. gov/28473875/

[11] Candi E, Tesauro M, Cardillo C, Lena AM, Schinzari F, Rodia G, et al. Metabolic profiling of visceral adipose tissue from obese subjects with or without metabolic syndrome. The Biochemical Journal. 2018;**475**(5): 1019-1035. Available from: https://pubmed.ncbi.nlm.nih.gov/29437994/

[12] Narath SH, Mautner SI, Svehlikova E, Schultes B, Pieber TR, et al. An untargeted metabolomics approach to characterize short-term and long-term metabolic changes after bariatric surgery. PLOS ONE. 2016;**11**(9):e0161425. https://doi.org/10.1371/journal.pone.0161425

[13] Sen P, Lamichhane S, Mathema VB, McGlinchey A, Dickens AM,

Khoomrung S, et al. Deep learning meets metabolomics: A methodological perspective. Briefings in Bioinformatics. 2021;**22**(2):1531-1542. Available from: https://pubmed.ncbi.nlm.nih.gov/32940335/

[14] Longitudinal Assessment of Bariatric Surgery (LABS) Consortium, Flum DR, Belle SH, King WC, Wahed AS, Berk P, et al. Perioperative safety in the longitudinal assessment of bariatric surgery. The New England Journal of Medicine. 2009;**361**(5): 445-454. Available from: https://pubmed.ncbi.nlm.nih.gov/19641201/

[15] Kim JH, Wolfe B. Bariatric/metabolic surgery: Short- and long-term safety. Current Atherosclerosis Reports. 2012;**14**(6):597-605. Available from: https://pubmed.ncbi.nlm.nih.gov/23054663/

[16] Chang SH, Stoll CRT, Song J, Varela JE, Eagon CJ, Colditz GA. The effectiveness and risks of bariatric surgery: An updated systematic review and meta-analysis, 2003-2012. JAMA Surgery. 2014;**149**(3):275-287. Available from: https://pubmed.ncbi.nlm.nih.gov/24352617/

[17] Aminian A, Brethauer SA, Kirwan JP, Kashyap SR, Burguera B, Schauer P. How safe is metabolic/diabetes surgery? Diabetes, Obesity & Metabolism. 2015;**17**(2):198-201. Available from: https://pubmed.ncbi.nlm.nih.gov/25352176/

[18] Phillips BT, Shikora SA. The history of metabolic and bariatric surgery: Development of standards for patient safety and efficacy. Metabolism. 2018;**79**:97-107. Available from: https://pubmed.ncbi.nlm.nih.gov/29307519/

[19] Arterburn D, Wellman R, Emiliano A, Smith SR, Odegaard AO, Murali S, et al. Comparative effectiveness and safety of bariatric procedures for weight loss: A PCORnet cohort study. Annals of Internal Medicine. 2018;**169**(11):741-750. Available from: https://pubmed.ncbi.nlm.nih.gov/30383139/

[20] Ghiassi S, Morton JM. Safety and efficacy of bariatric and metabolic surgery. Current Obesity Reports. 2020;**9**(2):159-164. Available from: https://pubmed.ncbi.nlm.nih.gov/32253662/

[21] Aminian A, Zajichek A, Arterburn DE, Wolski KE, Brethauer SA, Schauer PR, et al. Association of metabolic surgery with major adverse cardiovascular outcomes in patients with type 2 diabetes and obesity. Journal of the American Medical Association. 2019;**322**(13):1271-1282. Available from: https://pubmed.ncbi.nlm.nih.gov/31475297/

[22] Goldberg I, Yang J, Nie L, Bates AT, Docimo S, Pryor AD, et al. Safety of bariatric surgery in patients older than 65 years. Surgery for Obesity and Related Diseases. 2019;**15**(8):1380-1387. Available from: https://pubmed.ncbi.nlm.nih.gov/31248793/

[23] Lopez EH, Munie S, Higgins R, Gould J, Kindel T. Morbidity and mortality after bariatric surgery in adolescents versus adults. The Journal of Surgical Research. 2020;**256**:180-186. Available from: https://pubmed.ncbi.nlm.nih.gov/32711173/

[24] Chen N, Zhou M, Dong X, Qu J, Gong F, Han Y, et al. Epidemiological and clinical characteristics of 99 cases of 2019 novel coronavirus pneumonia in Wuhan, China: A descriptive study. Lancet (London, England). 2020;**395**(10223):507-513. Available from: https://pubmed.ncbi.nlm.nih.gov/32007143/

[25] Petrilli CM, Jones SA, Yang J, Rajagopalan H, O'Donnell L, Chernyak Y, et al. Factors associated with hospital admission and critical illness among 5279 people with coronavirus disease 2019 in New York City: Prospective cohort study. BMJ 2020;**369**:m1966. Available from: https://pubmed.ncbi.nlm.nih.gov/32444366/

[26] Singhal R, Tahrani AA, Ludwig C, Mahawar K, Abou-Mrad-Fricquegnon A, Alasfur A, et al. Global 30-day outcomes after bariatric surgery during the COVID-19 pandemic (GENEVA): An international cohort study. The Lancet Diabetes and Endocrinology. 2021;**9**(1):7-9. Available from: http://www.thelancet.com/article/S2213858720303752/fulltext

[27] Singhal R, Ludwig C, Rudge G, Gkoutos GV, Tahrani A, Mahawar K, et al. 30-day morbidity and mortality of bariatric surgery during the COVID-19 pandemic: A multinational cohort study of 7704 patients from 42 countries. Obesity Surgery. 2021;**31**(10):4272-4288. Available from: https://pubmed.ncbi.nlm.nih.gov/34328624/

[28] Singhal R, Wiggins T, Super J, Alqahtani A, Nadler EP, Ludwig C, et al. 30-day morbidity and mortality of bariatric metabolic surgery in adolescence during the COVID-19 pandemic—The GENEVA study. Pediatric Obesity. 2021 Dec;**16**(12):e12832. DOI: 10.1111/ijpo.12832. Epub 2021 Jul 8

[29] Singhal R, Cardoso VR, Wiggins T, Super J, Ludwig C, Gkoutos GV, et al. 30-day morbidity and mortality of sleeve gastrectomy, Roux-en-Y gastric bypass and one anastomosis gastric bypass: A propensity score-matched analysis of the GENEVA data. International Journal of Obesity. 2021;**46**(4):750-757. Available from: https://www.nature.com/articles/s41366-021-01048-1

[30] Singhal R, Omar I, Madhok B. et al. Safety of bariatric surgery in ≥ 65-year-old patients during the COVID-19 pandemic. Obesity Surgery. 2022;**32**:1-13. https://doi.org/10.1007/s11695-022-06067-z

[31] Elfanagely O, Toyoda Y, Othman S, Mellia JA, Basta M, Liu T, et al. Machine learning and surgical outcomes prediction: A systematic review. The Journal of Surgical Research. 2021;**264**:346-361. Available from: https://pubmed.ncbi.nlm.nih.gov/33848833/

[32] Henn J, Buness A, Schmid M, Kalff JC, Matthaei H. Machine learning to guide clinical decision-making in abdominal surgery—A systematic literature review. Langenbeck's Archives of Surgery. 2022;**407**(1):51-61. Available from: https://pubmed.ncbi.nlm.nih.gov/34716472/

[33] Stam WT, Goedknegt LK, Ingwersen EW, Schoonmade LJ, Bruns ERJ, Daams F. The prediction of surgical complications using artificial intelligence in patients undergoing major abdominal surgery: A systematic review. Surgery. 2022;**171**(4):1014-1021

[34] Cao Y, Fang X, Ottosson J, Näslund E, Stenberg E. A comparative study of machine learning algorithms in predicting severe complications after bariatric surgery. Journal of Clinical Medicine. 2019;**8**(5):668. Available from: https://pubmed.ncbi.nlm.nih.gov/31083643/

[35] Cao Y, Montgomery S, Ottosson J, Näslund E, Stenberg E. Deep learning neural networks to predict serious complications after bariatric surgery: Analysis of scandinavian obesity surgery registry data. JMIR Medical Informatics. 2020;**8**(5):e15992. DOI: 10.2196/15992. PMID: 32383681. PMCID: 7244994

[36] Razzaghi T, Safro I, Ewing J, Sadrfaridpour E, Scott JD. Predictive models for bariatric surgery risks with imbalanced medical datasets. Annals of Operations Research. 2019;**280**(1-2):1-18. Available from: https://link.springer.com/article/10.1007/s10479-019-03156-8

[37] Charles-Nelson A, Lazzati A, Katsahian S. Analysis of trajectories of care after bariatric surgery using data mining method and health administrative information systems. Obesity Surgery. 2020;**30**(6):2206-2216. Available from: https://pubmed.ncbi.nlm.nih.gov/32030617/

[38] Wise ES, Amateau SK, Ikramuddin S, Leslie DB. Prediction of thirty-day morbidity and mortality after laparoscopic sleeve gastrectomy: Data from an artificial neural network. Surgical Endoscopy. 2020;**34**(8):3590-3596. Available from: https://pubmed.ncbi.nlm.nih.gov/31571034/

[39] Sheikhtaheri A, Orooji A, Pazouki A, Beitollahi M. A clinical decision support system for predicting the early complications of one-anastomosis gastric bypass surgery. Obesity Surgery. 2019;**29**(7):2276-2286. Available from: https://pubmed.ncbi.nlm.nih.gov/31028626/

[40] Dang JT, Switzer N, Delisle M, Laffin M, Gill R, Birch DW, et al. Predicting venous thromboembolism following laparoscopic bariatric surgery: Development of the BariClot tool using the MBSAQIP database. Surgical Endoscopy. 2019;**33**(3):821-831. Available from: https://pubmed.ncbi.nlm.nih.gov/30003351/

[41] Nudel J, Bishara AM, de Geus SWL, Patil P, Srinivasan J, Hess DT, et al. Development and validation of machine learning models to predict gastrointestinal leak and venous thromboembolism after weight loss surgery: An analysis of the MBSAQIP database. Surgical Endoscopy. 2021;**35**(1):182-191. Available from: https://pubmed.ncbi.nlm.nih.gov/31953733/

[42] Liew PL, Lee YC, Lin YC, Lee TS, Lee WJ, Wang W, et al. Comparison of artificial neural networks with logistic regression in prediction of gallbladder disease among obese patients. Digestive and Liver Disease. 2007;**39**(4):356-362. Available from: https://pubmed.ncbi.nlm.nih.gov/17317348/

[43] Cruz MR, Martins C, Dias J, Pinto JS. A validation of an intelligent decision-making support system for the nutrition diagnosis of bariatric surgery patients. JMIR Medical Informatics. 2014;**2**(2):e8. Available from: http://www.ncbi.nlm.nih.gov/pubmed/25601419

[44] Segovia-Miranda F, Morales-Navarrete H, Kücken M, Moser V, Seifert S, Repnik U, et al. Three-dimensional spatially resolved geometrical and functional models of human liver tissue reveal new aspects of NAFLD progression. Nature Medicine. 2019;**25**(12):1885-1893. Available from: https://pubmed.ncbi.nlm.nih.gov/31792455/

[45] Zhang Q, Dong J, Zhou D, Liu F. Comparative risk of fracture for bariatric procedures in patients with obesity: A systematic review and Bayesian network meta-analysis: Bariatric procedures and fracture risk. International Journal of Surgery. 2020;**75**:13-23. Available from: https://pubmed.ncbi.nlm.nih.gov/31978646/

[46] Gloy VL, Briel M, Bhatt DL, Kashyap SR, Schauer PR, Mingrone G, Bucher HC, Nordmann AJ. Bariatric surgery versus non-surgical treatment for obesity: A systematic review and

meta-analysis of randomised controlled trials. BMJ. 2013 Oct 22;**347**:f5934. DOI: 10.1136/bmj.f5934. PMID: 24149519. PMD: PMC3806364

[47] Cheng J, Gao J, Shuai X, Wang G, Tao K. The comprehensive summary of surgical versus non-surgical treatment for obesity: A systematic review and meta-analysis of randomized controlled trials. Oncotarget. 2016;**7**(26):39216. Available from: /pmc/articles/PMC5129927/

[48] Heo YS, Park JM, Kim YJ, Kim SM, Park DJ, Lee SK, et al. Bariatric surgery versus conventional therapy in obese Korea patients: A multicenter retrospective cohort study. Journal of the Korean Surgical Society. 2012;**83**(6): 335-342. Available from: https://pubmed.ncbi.nlm.nih.gov/23230551/

[49] Park JY, Heo Y, Kim YJ, Park JM, Kim SM, Park DJ, et al. Long-term effect of bariatric surgery versus conventional therapy in obese Korean patients: A multicenter retrospective cohort study. Annals of Surgical Treatment and Research. 2019;**96**(6):283-289. Available from: https://pubmed.ncbi.nlm.nih.gov/31183332/

[50] Greenstein RJ, Rabner JG, Taler Y. Bariatric surgery vs. conventional dieting in the morbidly obese. Obesity Surgery. 1994;**4**(1):16-23. Available from: https://pubmed.ncbi.nlm.nih.gov/10742758/

[51] Martins C, Strømmen M, Stavne OA, Nossum R, Mårvik R, Kulseng B. Bariatric surgery versus lifestyle interventions for morbid obesity—Changes in body weight, risk factors and comorbidities at 1 year. Obesity Surgery. 2011;**21**(7):841-849. Available from: https://pubmed.ncbi.nlm.nih.gov/20379796/

[52] Ribaric G, Buchwald JN, McGlennon TW. Diabetes and weight in comparative studies of bariatric surgery vs conventional medical therapy: A systematic review and meta-analysis. Obesity Surgery. 2014;**24**(3):437-455. Available from: https://pubmed.ncbi.nlm.nih.gov/24374842/

[53] Bond DS, Phelan S, Leahey TM, Hill JO, Wing RR. Weight-loss maintenance in successful weight losers: Surgical vs non-surgical methods. International Journal of Obesity. 2009;**33**(1):173-180. Available from: https://pubmed.ncbi.nlm.nih.gov/19050676/

[54] Karpińska IA, Kulawik J, Pisarska-Adamczyk M, Wysocki M, Pędziwiatr M, Major P. Is it possible to predict weight loss after bariatric surgery?—External validation of predictive models. Obesity Surgery. 2021;**31**(7):2994-3004. Available from: https://link.springer.com/article/10.1007/s11695-021-05341-w

[55] Lee YC, Lee WJ, Lee TS, Lin YC, Wang W, Liew PL, et al. Prediction of successful weight reduction after bariatric surgery by data mining technologies. Obesity Surgery. 2007;**17**(9):1235-1241. Available from: https://pubmed.ncbi.nlm.nih.gov/18074500/

[56] Giraud-Carrier C, Pixton B, Rocha RA. Bariatric surgery performance: A predictive informatics case study. Intelligent Data Analysis. 2009;**13**(5):741-754

[57] Modaresnezhad M, Vahdati A, Nemati H, Ardestani A, Sadri F. A rule-based semantic approach for data integration, standardization and dimensionality reduction utilizing the UMLS: Application to predicting bariatric surgery outcomes. Computers in Biology and Medicine. 2019;**106**: 84-90. Available from: https://pubmed.ncbi.nlm.nih.gov/30708220/

[58] Perez-Leighton CE, Hamm JD, Shechter A, Tamura S, Laferrère B, Pi-Sunyer X, et al. Preoperative liking and wanting for sweet beverages as predictors of body weight loss after roux-en-Y gastric bypass and sleeve gastrectomy. International Journal of Obesity. 2020;**44**(6):1350-1359. Available from: https://pubmed.ncbi.nlm.nih.gov/31641214/

[59] Piaggi P, Lippi C, Fierabracci P, Maffei M, Calderone A, Mauri M, et al. Artificial neural networks in the outcome prediction of adjustable gastric banding in obese women. PLoS One. 2010 Oct;**27**;5(10):e13624. DOI: 10.1371/journal.pone.0013624. PMID: 21048960; PMCID: PMC2965091

[60] Celik S, Sohail A, Arif F, Özdemir A. Benchmarking coefficients for forecasting weight loss after sleeve gastrectomy biomedical engineering. Biomedical Engineering: Applications, Basis and Communications. 2020;**32**(1):14, 2050004. DOI: 10.4015/S1016237220500040

[61] Wise ES, Hocking KM, Kavic SM. Prediction of excess weight loss after laparoscopic roux-en-Y gastric bypass: Data from an artificial neural network. Surgical Endoscopy. 2016;**30**(2):480-488. Available from: https://pubmed.ncbi.nlm.nih.gov/26017908/

[62] Choudhury RA, Murayama KM, Abt PL, Glick HA, Naji A, Williams NN, et al. Roux-en-Y gastric bypass compared with aggressive diet and exercise therapy for morbidly obese patients awaiting renal transplant: A decision analysis. Surgery for Obesity and Related Diseases. 2014;**10**(1):79-87. Available from: https://pubmed.ncbi.nlm.nih.gov/24139923/

[63] De Luca M, Angrisani L, Himpens J, Busetto L, Scopinaro N, Weiner R, et al. Indications for surgery for obesity and weight-related diseases: Position statements from the International Federation for the Surgery of obesity and metabolic disorders (IFSO). Obesity Surgery. 2016;**26**(8):1659-1696. Available from: https://pubmed.ncbi.nlm.nih.gov/27412673/

[64] Ikramuddin S, Korner J, Lee WJ, Connett JE, Inabnet WB, Billington CJ, et al. Roux-en-Y gastric bypass vs intensive medical management for the control of type 2 diabetes, hypertension, and hyperlipidemia: The diabetes surgery study randomized clinical trial. Journal of the American Medical Association. 2013;**309**(21):2240-2249. Available from: https://pubmed.ncbi.nlm.nih.gov/23736733/

[65] Jakobsen GS, Småstuen MC, Sandbu R, Nordstrand N, Hofsø D, Lindberg M, et al. Association of bariatric surgery vs medical obesity treatment with long-term medical complications and obesity-related comorbidities. JAMA—Journal of the American Medical Association. 2018;**319**(3):291-301

[66] Mingrone G, Panunzi S, De Gaetano A, Guidone C, Iaconelli A, Nanni G, et al. Bariatric-metabolic surgery versus conventional medical treatment in obese patients with type 2 diabetes: 5 year follow-up of an open-label, single-centre, randomised controlled trial. Lancet. 2015;**386**(9997):964-973. Available from: http://www.thelancet.com/article/S0140673615000756/fulltext

[67] Mingrone G, Panunzi S, De Gaetano A, Guidone C, Iaconelli A, Capristo E, et al. Metabolic surgery versus conventional medical therapy in patients with type 2 diabetes: 10-year follow-up of an open-label, single-Centre, randomised controlled trial.

Lancet. 2021;**397**(10271):293-304. Available from: http://www.thelancet.com/article/S0140673620326490/fulltext

[68] Schauer PR, Kashyap SR, Wolski K, Brethauer SA, Kirwan JP, Pothier CE, et al. Bariatric surgery versus intensive medical therapy in obese patients with diabetes. The New England Journal of Medicine. 2012;**366**(17):1567-1576. Available from: https://pubmed.ncbi.nlm.nih.gov/22449319/

[69] Schauer PR, Bhatt DL, Kirwan JP, Wolski K, Aminian A, Brethauer SA, et al. Bariatric surgery versus intensive medical therapy for diabetes—5-year outcomes. The New England Journal of Medicine. 2017;**376**(7):641-651. Available from:. DOI: https://www.nejm.org/doi/10.1056/NEJMoa1600869

[70] Rubino F. From bariatric to metabolic surgery: Definition of a new discipline and implications for clinical practice. Current Atherosclerosis Reports. 2013;**369**(15):7. https://doi.org/10.1007/s11883-013-0369-x

[71] Rubino F, Nathan DM, Eckel RH, Schauer PR, Alberti KGMM, Zimmet PZ, et al. Metabolic surgery in the treatment algorithm for type 2 diabetes: A joint statement by international diabetes organizations. Diabetes Care. 2016;**39**(6):861-877. Available from: https://pubmed.ncbi.nlm.nih.gov/27222544/

[72] Cao Y, Raoof M, Szabo E, Ottosson J, Näslund I. Using Bayesian networks to predict long-term health-related quality of life and comorbidity after bariatric surgery: A study based on the Scandinavian obesity surgery registry. Journal of Clinical Medicine. 2020;**9**(6):1895. Available from: https://pubmed.ncbi.nlm.nih.gov/32560424/

[73] van Loon SLM, Deneer R, Nienhuijs SW, Wilbik A, Kaymak U, van Riel N, et al. Metabolic health index (MHI): Assessment of comorbidity in bariatric patients based on biomarkers. Obesity Surgery. 2020;**30**(2):714-724. Available from: https://pubmed.ncbi.nlm.nih.gov/31724117/

[74] Lee WJ, Hur KY, Lakadawala M, Kasama K, Wong SKH, Lee YC. Gastrointestinal metabolic surgery for the treatment of diabetic patients: A multi-institutional international study. Journal of Gastrointestinal Surgery. 2012;**16**(1):45-52. Available from: https://pubmed.ncbi.nlm.nih.gov/22042564/

[75] Lee WJ, Chong K, Chen JC, Ser KH, Lee YC, Tsou JJ, et al. Predictors of diabetes remission after bariatric surgery in Asia. Asian Journal of Surgery. 2012;**35**(2):67-73. Available from: https://pubmed.ncbi.nlm.nih.gov/22720861/

[76] Lee YC, Lee WJ, Liew PL. Predictors of remission of type 2 diabetes mellitus in obese patients after gastrointestinal surgery. Obesity Research & Clinical Practice. 2013 Dec;7(6):e494-500. DOI: 10.1016/j.orcp.2012.08.190. PMID: 24308892

[77] Aron-Wisnewsky J, Sokolovska N, Liu Y, Comaneshter DS, Vinker S, Pecht T, et al. The advanced-DiaRem score improves prediction of diabetes remission 1 year post-roux-en-Y gastric bypass. Diabetologia. 2017;**60**(10):1892-1902. Available from: https://pubmed.ncbi.nlm.nih.gov/28733906/

[78] Debédat J, Sokolovska N, Coupaye M, Panunzi S, Chakaroun R, Genser L, et al. Long-term relapse of type 2 diabetes after Roux-en-Y gastric bypass: Prediction and clinical relevance. Diabetes Care. 1 October 2018;**41**(10):2086-2095. https://doi.org/10.2337/dc18-0567

[79] Aminian A, Brethauer SA, Kashyap SR, Kirwan JP, Schauer PR. DiaRem score: External validation. The Lancet Diabetes and Endocrinology. 2014;**2**(1):12-13. Available from: http://www.thelancet.com/article/S221385871370202X/fulltext

[80] Park JY. Prediction of type 2 diabetes remission after bariatric or metabolic surgery. Journal of Obesity & Metabolic Syndrome. 2018;**27**(4):213-222

[81] Craig Wood G, Horwitz D, Still CD, Mirshahi T, Benotti P, Parikh M, et al. Performance of the DiaRem score for predicting diabetes remission in two health systems following bariatric surgery procedures in Hispanic and non-Hispanic white patients. Obesity Surgery. 2018;**28**(1):61. Available from: /pmc/articles/PMC5736407/

[82] Aminian A, Zajichek A, Arterburn DE, Wolski KE, Brethauer SA, Schauer PR, et al. Predicting 10-year risk of end-organ complications of type 2 diabetes with and without metabolic surgery: A machine learning approach. Diabetes Care. 2020;**43**(4):852-859. Available from: https://pubmed.ncbi.nlm.nih.gov/32029638/

[83] Pedersen HK, Gudmundsdottir V, Pedersen MK, Brorsson C, Brunak S, Gupta R. Ranking factors involved in diabetes remission after bariatric surgery using machine-learning integrating clinical and genomic biomarkers. NPJ Genomic Medicine. 2016 Oct 26;1:8,16035. DOI: 10.1038/npjgenmed.2016.35. PMID: 29263820; PMCID: PMC5685313

[84] Lassailly G, Caiazzo R, Ntandja-Wandji LC, Gnemmi V, Baud G, Verkindt H, et al. Bariatric surgery provides long-term resolution of nonalcoholic steatohepatitis and regression of fibrosis. Gastroenterology. 2020;**159**(4):1290-1301.e5. Available from: https://pubmed.ncbi.nlm.nih.gov/32553765/

[85] Zhang C, Yang M. Current options and future directions for NAFLD and NASH treatment. Int J Mol Sci. 2021 Jul 15;22(14):7571. DOI: 10.3390/ijms22147571. PMID: 34299189; PMCID: PMC8306701

[86] Codjia T, Rebibo L, François A, Lagnel C, Huet E, Bekri S, et al. Evolution of non-alcoholic fatty liver disease (NAFLD) biomarkers in response to weight loss 1 year after bariatric surgery-a post hoc analysis of the FibroTest prospective study. Obesity Surgery. 2021;**31**(8):3548-3556. Available from: https://pubmed.ncbi.nlm.nih.gov/33844174/

[87] Sowa JP, Heider D, Bechmann LP, Gerken G, Hoffmann D, Canbay A. Novel algorithm for non-invasive assessment of fibrosis in NAFLD. PLoS One. 2013 Apr 30;**8**(4):e62439. DOI: 10.1371/journal.pone.0062439. PMID: 23638085; PMCID: PMC3640062

[88] Uehara D, Hayashi Y, Seki Y, Kakizaki S, Horiguchi N, Tojima H, et al. Non-invasive prediction of non-alcoholic steatohepatitis in Japanese patients with morbid obesity by artificial intelligence using rule extraction technology. World Journal of Hepatology. 2018;**10**(12):934-943. Available from: https://pubmed.ncbi.nlm.nih.gov/30631398/

[89] Oria HE, Moorehead MK. Updated bariatric analysis and reporting outcome system (BAROS). Surgery for Obesity and Related Diseases. 2009;**5**(1):60-66. Available from: https://pubmed.ncbi.nlm.nih.gov/19161935/

[90] Hörchner R, Tuinebreijer W, Kelder H. Quality-of-life assessment of morbidly obese patients who have undergone a Lap-Band® operation:

2-Year follow-up study: Is the MOS SF-36 a useful instrument to measure quality of life in morbidly obese patients? Obesity Surgery. 2001;**11**(2):212-218. Available from:. DOI: https://link.springer.com/article/10.1381/096089201321577901

[91] Lechaux D, Le Foll D, Rascle O. Weight loss and quality of life after sleeve gastrectomy or one-anastomosis gastric bypass: Results of a prospective study of 120 women with morbid obesity. Obesity Surgery. 2020;**30**(7):2828-2831. Available from: https://link.springer.com/article/10.1007/s11695-020-04442-2

[92] Fiorani C, Coles SR, Kulendran M, McGlone ER, Reddy M, Khan OA. Long-term quality of life outcomes after laparoscopic sleeve gastrectomy and roux-en-Y gastric bypass—A comparative study. Obesity Surgery. 2021;**31**(3):1376-1380. Available from: https://link.springer.com/article/10.1007/s11695-020-05049-3

[93] Cao Y, Raoof M, Montgomery S, Ottosson J, Näslund I. Predicting long-term health-related quality of life after bariatric surgery using a conventional neural network: A study based on the Scandinavian obesity surgery registry. Journal of Clinical Medicine. 2019;**8**(12):2149. Available from: https://pubmed.ncbi.nlm.nih.gov/31817385/

[94] Małczak P, Mizera M, Lee Y, Pisarska-Adamczyk M, Wysocki M, Bała MM, et al. Quality of life after bariatric surgery-a systematic review with Bayesian network meta-analysis. Obesity Surgery. 2021;**31**(12):5213-5223. Available from: https://pubmed.ncbi.nlm.nih.gov/34633614/

[95] Lam K, Chen J, Wang Z, Iqbal FM, Darzi A, Lo B, et al. Machine learning for technical skill assessment in surgery: A systematic review. npj Digital Medicine. 2022;**5**(1):1-16. Available from: https://www.nature.com/articles/s41746-022-00566-0

[96] Twinanda AP, De Mathelin M, Padoy N. Fisher kernel based task boundary retrieval in laparoscopic database with single video query. In: Medical Image Computing and Computer-Assisted Intervention – MICCAI 2014: 17th International Conference, Boston, MA, USA, September 14-18, 2014, Proceedings, Part III). Series: Lecture Notes in Computer Science 8675 Image Processing, Computer Vision, Pattern Recognition, and Graphics. Springer International Publishing, Springer Verlag; 2014. ISBN: 978-3-319-10442-3, 978-3-319-10443-0 pp. 409-416. Available from: https://pubmed.ncbi.nlm.nih.gov/25320826/

[97] Twinanda AP, Yengera G, Mutter D, Marescaux J, Padoy N. RSDNet: Learning to predict remaining surgery duration from laparoscopic videos without manual annotations. IEEE Transactions on Medical Imaging. 2019;**38**(4):1069-1078. Available from: https://pubmed.ncbi.nlm.nih.gov/30371356/

[98] Hashimoto DA, Rosman G, Witkowski ER, Stafford C, Navarette-Welton AJ, Rattner DW, et al. Computer vision analysis of intraoperative video: Automated recognition of operative steps in laparoscopic sleeve gastrectomy. Annals of Surgery. 2019;**270**(3):414-421. Available from: https://pubmed.ncbi.nlm.nih.gov/31274652/

[99] Derathé A, Reche F, Moreau-Gaudry A, Jannin P, Gibaud B, Voros S. Predicting the quality of surgical exposure using spatial and procedural features from laparoscopic videos. International Journal of Computer Assisted Radiology and Surgery. 2020;**15**(1):59-67. Available

from: https://pubmed.ncbi.nlm.nih.gov/31673963/

[100] Heremans ERM, Chen AS, Wang X, Cheng J, Xu F, Martinez AE, et al. Artificial neural network-based automatic detection of food intake for neuromodulation in treating obesity and diabetes. Obesity Surgery. 2020;**30**(7):2547-2557. Available from: https://pubmed.ncbi.nlm.nih.gov/32103435/

[101] Ademi Z, Bucher HC, Glinz D, et al. Bariatric surgery vs. conservative treatment for obesity and overweight. Swiss Medical Board. 2016. DOI: 10.13140/RG.2.1.2195.8804. Available from: https://www.researchgate.net/publication/299599772

[102] Borisenko O, Adam D, Funch-Jensen P, Ahmed AR, Zhang R, Colpan Z, et al. Bariatric surgery can Lead to net cost savings to health care systems: Results from a comprehensive European decision analytic model. Obesity Surgery. 2015;**25**(9):1559-1568. Available from: https://pubmed.ncbi.nlm.nih.gov/25639648/

[103] Borisenko O, Lukyanov V, Debergh I, Dillemans B. Cost-effectiveness analysis of bariatric surgery for morbid obesity in Belgium. Journal of Medical Economics. 2018;**21**(4):365-373. Available from: https://pubmed.ncbi.nlm.nih.gov/29271279/

[104] Faria GR, Preto JR, Costa-Maia J. Gastric bypass is a cost-saving procedure: Results from a comprehensive markov model. Obesity Surgery. 2013;**23**(4):460-466

[105] Wang F, Casalino LP, Khullar D. Deep learning in medicine—Promise, progress, and challenges. JAMA Internal Medicine. 2019;**179**(3):293-294. Available from: https://jamanetwork.com/journals/jamainternalmedicine/fullarticle/2718342

[106] Parikh RB, Teeple S, Navathe AS. Addressing bias in artificial intelligence in health care. Journal of the American Medical Association. 2019;**322**(24):2377-2378. Available from: https://jamanetwork.com/journals/jama/fullarticle/2756196

[107] Price WN, Gerke S, Cohen IG. Potential liability for physicians using artificial intelligence. JAMA—Journal of the American Medical Association. American Medical Association. 2019;**322**:1765-1766. Available from: https://pubmed.ncbi.nlm.nih.gov/31584609/

[108] Khullar D, Casalino LP, Qian Y, Lu Y, Krumholz HM, Aneja S. Perspectives of patients about artificial intelligence in health care. JAMA Network Open. 2022;**5**(5):e2210309-e2210309. Available from: https://jamanetwork.com/journals/jamanetworkopen/fullarticle/2791851

[109] Bellini V, Valente M, Turetti M, Del Rio P, Saturno F, Maffezzoni M, et al. Current applications of artificial intelligence in bariatric surgery. Obesity Surgery. 2022;**1**:1-17. Available from: https://link.springer.com/article/10.1007/s11695-022-06100-1

Chapter 7

Gut Microbiota and Bariatric Surgery

Natalia Bastón-Paz, Manuel Ponce-Alonso, José Avendaño, María Garriga and Rosa del Campo

Abstract

The gut microbiota comprise all the living organisms in our intestine. Microbiota has key roles in metabolic homeostasis, digestion and nutrient metabolism protection against pathogens or modulation of the immune system. Advances in techniques such as metagenomics or metabolomics have expanded our knowledge of the intestinal ecosystem. Beyond genetic, behavioral, or environmental factors, alterations of gut microbiota parameters such as composition, diversity, or metabolites including short-chain fatty acids, have shown to be associated with cardiovascular comorbidities. In this chapter, we described the role of the gut microbiota in obesity and type 2 diabetes pathophysiology, and the changes it undergoes during bariatric surgery, as well as explored the possibilities of modifying the microbiome to obtain potential clinical benefits.

Keywords: gut microbiota, obesity, type 2 diabetes, bariatric surgery, diet, probiotics, fecal microbiota transplant

1. Introduction

The human organism is a complex biological system composed of cells belonging to three domains: Eukarya, Bacteria, and Archaea, in addition to viruses [1, 2]. The microbiome has been considered as the last human organ [1] and can be defined as the whole genomic and metabolomic content of the microbial community that coexists and interacts with our cells [3]. The gut microbiota, the most complex and abundant microbiome [4], is the focus of this chapter because of its direct relationship with obesity and bariatric surgery.

The gut microbiota has traditionally been studied by culturing, with the aim of identifying and characterizing single isolated microorganisms related to acute or chronic infections [5]. Although culturing techniques are improving with various strategies [6, 7], their resolution is insufficient because most bacteria are uncultivable. Today, microbiota studies are focusing on the overall ecosystem, not only individual microorganisms; and to address the real effect of microbiota colonization on human health over prolonged periods.

Knowledge of the human microbiome has exploded in the last two decades due to the development of genomic strategies based on marker genes such as 16S ribosomal

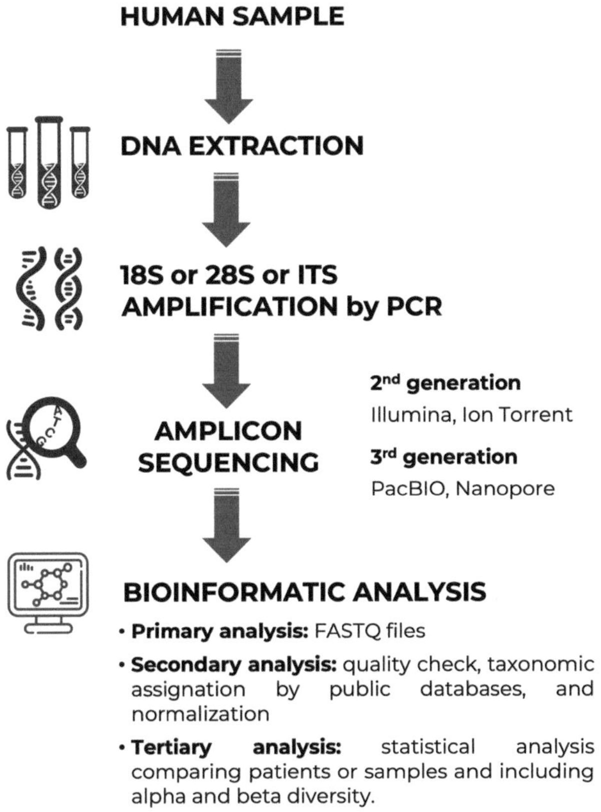

Figure 1.
Schematic representation of the usual workflow in the study of the bacterial composition in a sample by NGS of 16S rDNA amplicons.

Approach	Data	Technology	Strength	Limitation
Biomarker sequencing (e.g., 16S rDNA)	Community composition	Next-generation sequencing	Cost-effective, semiquantitative, achieves genus level resolution	Shorts reads may make accurate classification difficult
Metagenomics	Generation of draft genomes, functional capacity, growth dynamics	Next-generation sequencing	Capacity for strain-level reconstruction, quantitative, allows for functional annotation with pathway predictions	Very costly, community coverage that may be relatively shallow in more complex assemblies
Metatranscriptomics (RNA sequencing)	Gene expression	Next-generation sequencing	Highly expressed genes are more likely than others to be detected, depletion of human transcripts is possible	Requires immediate preservation or processing of fresh or snap-frozen intestinal specimens

Approach	Data	Technology	Strength	Limitation
Metaproteomics	Protein expression	Liquid or gas chromatography–mass spectrometry	Primarily detects dominant proteins	No removal of host-derived proteins
Metabolomics	Metabolic productivity	Liquid or gas chromatography–mass spectrometry or magnetic resonance spectroscopy	Semiquantitative, can be targeted or untargeted	Metabolite identification are platform- and database-dependent. Detects metabolites that may originate from microbes, diet, or host

Table 1.
Summary of the most common techniques available for the study of the microbiome.

DNA (rDNA), and massive sequencing techniques, also known as next-generation sequencing (NGS) (**Figure 1**). Multi-omics technologies, including metagenome, metatranscriptome, metaproteome, and metabolome approaches provide valuable information on microbial functions [8]. The high potential of combining various "omics" techniques to analyze host-microorganism interactions allows us to dissect the molecular mechanisms by which microbiomes influence human health. A summary of the characteristics of each technique is shown in **Table 1**. Bioinformatics analysis of these big data allows us to characterize the ecological biodiversity of a given microbial community and draw conclusions [9]. Nonetheless, this field of research is beyond the scope of this chapter.

2. The importance of sampling

Microbiota composition is typically studied in biological samples, such as stool, mucosal biopsy, intestinal aspirate, luminal brushing, etc.; for population studies, however, sampling should be noninvasive and performed mainly in healthy conditions. In practice, although fecal samples are the most used as a representation of the intestinal tract, significant differences have been demonstrated among the mucosal microbiota of each intestinal anatomic region [10, 11]. Its main limitations are that feces also contain DNA from microorganisms ingested with food, which are not part of our microbiota; that we are not able to differentiate between living and dead microorganisms; and given that diet causes fluctuations in its composition, longitudinal sampling is required to decipher the real core of the native microbiota.

After deposition, strict anaerobic bacteria begin to lose viability after contact with oxygen, an irrelevant factor if DNA techniques are used. However, numerous studies have demonstrated the influence on the results of collection, transport, storage, and processing of the samples [12]. All samples belonging to the same study should be collected, preserved, and processed simultaneously and identically, to minimize any source of variability [13]. As a rule, recommendations on feces collection consist of using a sterile container with a screw cap, which should be transported without delay to the processing center and frozen as soon as possible at −80°C, although it is also acceptable to perform a first freeze at higher temperatures (as low as −20°C). Freezing prevents changes in microbial communities until nucleic acid extraction can be performed, which is crucial for RNA analysis because it is more easily degraded than DNA in freeze–thaw cycles. Therefore, optimizing sampling methods should not be ignored. Future sampling procedures should include reducing invasiveness, performing non-cross-contamination sampling, and minimizing disturbance to normal intestinal physiology [12].

3. Gut microbiota composition

The parameters that help us to characterize the microbiome have been classically used in ecology and can be separated into those related to alpha diversity, which is a measure of microbiome diversity that allows us to define the total number of species and their relative contribution applicable to a single sample (Shannon or Chao1 indexes, i.e.); and beta diversity, which is a measure of similarity or dissimilarity between two communities, allowing us to compare ecosystems of different subjects or times (Bray-Curtis or UniFrac metrics, i.e.) [14, 15].

Currently, there is no consensus on the "normal" composition of the microbiota or universal cutoff points for classifying a microbiome as healthy or pathological according to the presence/absence or abundance of certain taxa in the overall ecosystem. It is generally considered that the greater the number of species present, and the more balanced the distribution of species, the healthier and more resilient the ecosystem [16].

The most dominant bacterial phyla of the human gut are Bacillota (formerly Firmicutes), Bacteroidota (formerly Bacteroidetes), Actinomycetota, and Pseudomonadota (formerly Proteobacteria), with *Bacteroides*, *Clostridium*, *Peptococcus*, *Bifidobacterium*, *Eubacterium*, *Ruminococcus*, *Faecalibacterium*, and *Peptostreptococcus* as the most abundant genera. Remarkably, *Bacteroides* family represents approximately 30% of the total bacteria, suggesting an important role in the global metabolism [4].

Beyond composition, the real impact of microbiota on human health is conditioned by their metabolism. This balanced host–microbe interaction can be defined as eubiosis, again habitually linked to high taxa diversity, high microbial gene richness, and stable microbiome functionality [8]. An imbalance in this functionality is defined as dysbiosis, a term typically used when the composition is different from that of healthy individuals; in our view, however, it is more a functional than compositional concept. This disturbance of gut microbiota can also modulate intestinal permeability as well as immune responses, favoring a proinflammatory state [5, 17, 18].

3.1 Factors affecting gut microbial composition

Several factors can influence microbiota composition. These factors include the mode of infant delivery and breastfeeding, diet, intake of antibiotics and other drugs, stress, disease, smoking, drinking, aging, and race, among others [18]. The main influencing factors are described below:

a. **Mode of infant delivery and breastfeeding.** The mode of delivery significantly affects gut colonization in newborns. Passage through the birth canal affords the neonate a microbiota like that of the mother's vagina, whereas for infants born via Cesarean-section, the microbiota resembles the mother's skin and environmental microorganisms [19, 20]. Breastfeeding also provides beneficial genera, such as *Bifidobacterium* and *Lactobacillus*, with a lower colonization rate by *Escherichia coli*, *Clostridium*, and *Bacteroides* [21, 22].

b. **Antibiotic exposure.** Various studies have shown both the short- and long-term impact of antibiotics on the gut microbiota [23, 24]. Among the short-term effects of antibiotic use reported are diarrhea and recurrent *Clostridioides difficile* infection [25]. The long-term effects include allergic conditions and obesity due to altered metabolic activity [26]. Lastly, systematic use of antibiotics can reduce bacterial species diversity, as well as selecting for antibiotic-resistant strains even after exposure has been eliminated.

c. **Diet.** Diet is the major factor conditioning gut microbiota composition. The Western diet has been associated with less bacterial alpha diversity compared with the Mediterranean diet and other diets with lower animal protein and high vegetable and fiber intake. Unlike the Western diet, which has been associated with a higher risk of obesity, diabetes, cancer, and cardiovascular disease due to high intakes of animal proteins, saturated fats, and simple sugars, the Mediterranean diet and plant-based diets prevent cardiovascular disease, reducing mortality risk and limiting weight gain. It has been reported that the consumption of a plant protein-based diet increases *Bifidobacterium* and *Lactobacillus* genera, as well as decreasing *Bacteroides* and *Clostridium* species [27, 28]. The intake of nondigestible carbohydrates, such as fiber and resistant starch, appears to have the highest impact of all nutritional components on gut microbiota composition, diversity, and metabolic profile [29].

d. **Lifestyle.** Lifestyle factors include physical activity, smoking, and the surrounding environment, to name a few. The individual's level of physical activity and their amount of exposure to pollutants are considered critical factors affecting microbiome composition [18]. Regarding physical activity, an active individual's microbiome possesses a greater abundance of beneficial bacteria, such as *Faecalibacterium*, *Roseburia*, and *Akkermansia* [30]. As for environmental exposure, certain pollutants have been associated with fewer taxa and higher numbers of *Bacteroides* and Bacillota [31]. Lastly, when comparing the gut microbiome of smokers with that of non-smokers and former smokers, that of smokers was found to be enriched with *Bacteroides* and reduced in Bacillota and Pseudomonadota [32].

4. Functions of gut microbiota

A mature, healthy gut microbiota has significant functions in the human body [4]: protection against pathogens by colonizing mucosal surfaces and production of various antimicrobial substances; development and modulation of the immune system; digestion and nutrient metabolism; control of cellular proliferation and differentiation; modification of insulin resistance and its secretion; and facilitation of dynamic communication between the gut and multiple organs [33, 34].

In Ref. to its role in enhancing the immune system, immunological immaturity is observed in germ-free and laboratory mice compared with wild mice, and humans residing on farms exhibit greater functional microbial diversity and a lower susceptibility to chronic inflammatory diseases [35]. The gut microbiota has also been described as an important immunoregulator of bone's remodeling processes [36, 37].

One of the most relevant roles of gut microbiota is the metabolism of dietary elements into bioactive food components. Indigestible carbohydrates are metabolized into short-chain fatty acids (SCFAs), such as acetic, propionic, and butyric acids, which are mainly produced due to fermentation by Bacillota, Bacteroidota, and other anaerobic bacteria. These compounds supply significant energy for intestinal epithelial cells, strengthen the mucosal barrier, contribute to intestinal homeostasis, and reduce inflammation [38]. Moreover, the gut microbiota participates in the biosynthesis of certain essential amino acids and vitamins and is involved in the synthesis of bile acids, cholesterol, and conjugated fatty acids [17]. On the other hand, other microbial derived-metabolites, such as trimethylamine N-oxide (TMAO), have been associated with cardiovascular disease [39].

Therefore, understanding the metabolic pathways of derived microbial compounds is crucial for establishing a link to the metabolism of the healthy host or to the pathogenesis of metabolic diseases.

5. Gut microbiota in obesity and type 2 diabetes mellitus

5.1 Obesity

Obesity is a complex and multifactorial disease with significant morbidity and mortality, and it is a major public health problem, particularly in the developed world [40]. Among the risk factors contributing to obesity (genetic, behavioral, socioeconomic, and environmental), the gut microbiota has been recognized as a major contributor [3]. More than 10 years ago, a differential gut bacterial composition linked to increased Bacillota and a reduction in Bacteroidota was demonstrated in genetically obese (ob/ob) mice compared with lean (ob/+) and wild-type (+/+) mice that had been fed with the same polysaccharide-enriched diet [41]. Moreover, after transplanting the obese and lean microbiomes to germ-free recipients, the phenotypes of the mouse donors were reproduced.

Numerous studies have been designed to identify significant differences in the bacterial gut microbiota composition between lean and obese individuals [42] and to describe the impact of the bariatric surgery approach to obesity [43]. Regarding bacteria, the Bacillota/Bacteroidota ratio has been discarded because it was proven ineffective as a differential marker of the microbiota in patients with obesity, given that an expansion of Bacillota leads to a proportional reduction of the other phyla [44]. The bariatric surgery approach will be discussed in a later section.

According to the following meta-analysis, which reviewed the composition of the gut microbiota in obese and non-obese individuals [45], no significant differences were found in alpha diversity. On the other hand, at the genus level, lower relative proportions of *Bifidobacterium* and *Eggerthella* (Actinomycetota) were observed in the obese group compared with the non-obese. The genera of *Acidaminococcus*, *Anaerococcus*, *Catenibacterium*, *Dialister*, *Dorea*, *Eubacterium*, *Megasphaera*, *Roseburia*, *Streptococcus* (all belonging to the Bacillota phylum), *Fusobacterium* (Fusobacteriota), *Prevotella* (Bacteroidota), *Escherichia-Shigella*, and *Sutterella* (Pseudomonadota) were significantly higher in the obese individuals. On the other hand, Verrucomicrobiota (*Akkermansia muciniphila*), *Faecalibacterium*, *Methanobrevibacter smithii*, and *Lactobacillus* species have a lower presence in obesity [46].

5.2 Type 2 diabetes mellitus

The etiology of type 2 diabetes mellitus (T2DM) involves a combination of genetic variants and environmental factors shared with obesity, in which most individuals are either overweight or obese. Insulin resistance is followed by a compensatory higher biosynthesis and insulin secretion.

Although there are some inconsistencies among studies, it appears that in the early stages of T2DM, before patients have been treated with anti-hyperglycemic drugs, the gut microbiota could have loss of butyrate-producing taxa, a marked reduction of *Akkermansia*, and an increase in proinflammatory bacterial genera such as Bacteroidota [47, 48].

The effects of metformin on the gut microbiota have been studied in patients with T2DM, demonstrating a higher relative abundance of *Akkermansia*, *Butyrivibrio*, *Bifidobacterium*, and *Megasphaera* compared with individuals without T2DM [49]. On the other hand, those with non-metformin treated T2DM had a higher relative abundance of Clostridiaceae and a lower abundance of *Enterococcus casseliflavus* compared with individuals without T2DM. The authors found significant associations between metformin intake and gut microbiota composition.

Additional studies [50, 51] have also observed shifts in gut microbiota in patients treated with metformin by increasing the abundance of *Akkermansia* and SCFA-producing bacteria, which activate intestinal gluconeogenesis, resulting in lower glycemic levels. *Akkermansia* participates in maintaining the cohesion of the mucin layer by reducing translocation of proinflammatory lipopolysaccharides and controlling fat deposition, adipose tissue metabolism, and glucose homeostasis. SCFAs, especially butyrate and propionate, trigger intestinal gluconeogenesis, benefitting glucose and energy homeostasis and reducing hepatic glucose production, appetite, and body weight.

Nevertheless, further large-scale studies are necessary to evaluate the interactions between the changes in gut microbiota and the effects of metformin to establish a potential target intervention from a microbiological perspective.

6. Impact of bariatric surgery on gut microbiota

As has been described throughout the present book, bariatric surgery (BS) is indicated as treatment for reducing body mass index (BMI) in severe obesity (BMI $\geq$40 Kg/m^2 or $\geq$ 35 Kg/m^2) with at least one obesity-related disease [52]. This surgery improves glycemic control because of weight loss and calorie restriction, along with increased insulin sensitivity and secretion [53]. Several changes in gut microbiota composition depending on the type of surgery have been observed.

The procedures vary, although the most common are sleeve gastrectomy (SG) and Roux-en-Y gastric bypass (RYGB). While SG is a restrictive approach based on stomach reduction, RYGB combines restrictive and malabsorptive approaches by reducing the stomach and anatomically reorganizing the biliary and digestive tracts [54]. These procedures alter the anatomy of the digestive and biliary tract, hormonal status, and the amount and choice of nutrients ingested, which could modify the composition of the microbiota and the quantity of several microbial metabolites [54, 55]. However, whether the evolution of the microbiota is the cause or the consequence of weight loss and improvement of obesity-related diseases (or whether the changes are more related to the specificities of the surgical procedure) remains to be determined.

One of the most relevant lines of research proposes to predict weight loss after BS by examining the basal composition of the gut microbiota. Previous studies have indicated that BS modifies the gut microbiota profiles [56, 57]. Changes in alpha diversity do not appear to be clear, but beta diversity analyses consistently show more profound changes for the RYGB approach with an expansion of the phylum

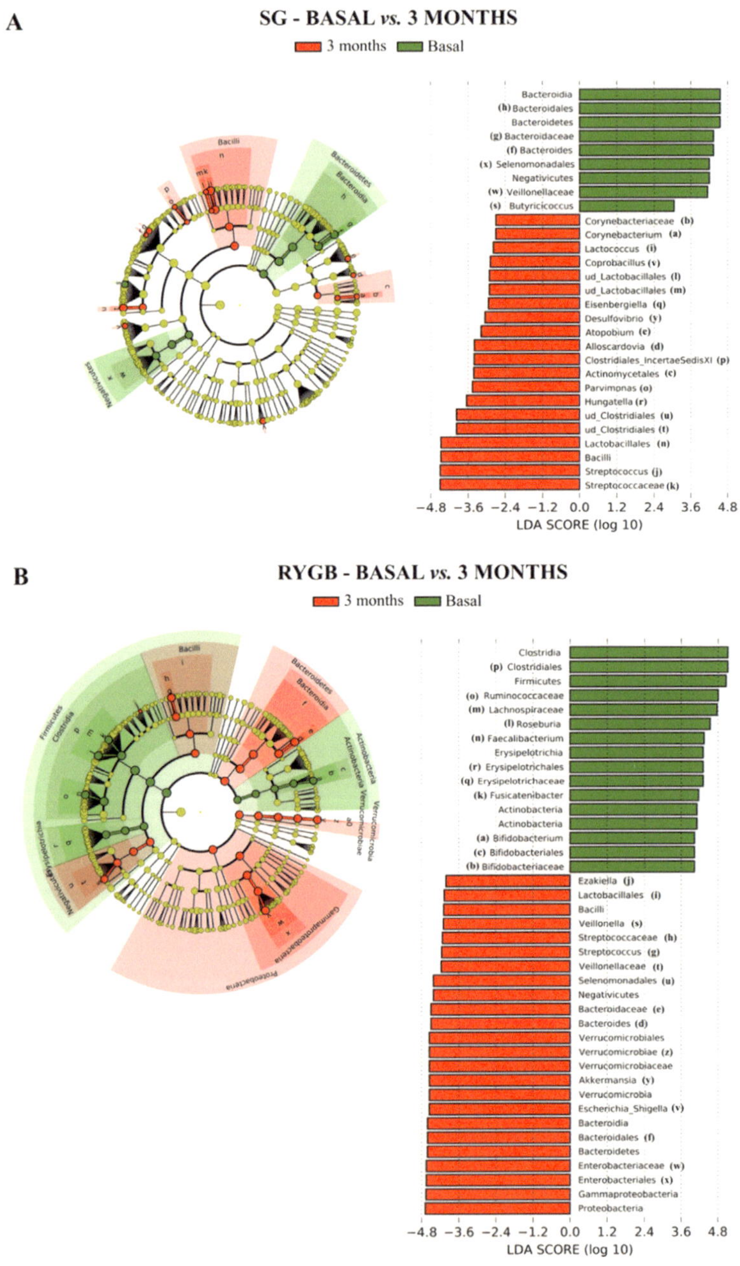

Figure 2.
Bacterial taxa with differential abundance according to linear effect size discriminant analysis (LEfSe). This representation shows the significant taxa ordered according to the magnitude of the differences [LDA score (only taxa with LDA > 4 are shown)]. A, comparison of microbiota composition between baseline and 3 months after SG surgery (n = 14). B, comparison of microbiota composition between baseline and 3 months after RYGB surgery (n = 26) (from: Salazar et al. [58]).

Pseudomonadota. Redistribution of the bile acid circuit, whose antibacterial activity limits the expansion of gamma-Proteobacteria in the small intestine, appears to be the main cause of the increase in the members of this phylum found in samples from patients undergoing RYGB [58].

In 2022, Salazar et al. [58] observed that BS caused a decrease in the genera *Roseburia*, *Faecalibacterium*, *Ruminococcus*, and *Bifidobacterium* and an increase in *Escherichia/Shigella* and *Akkermansia*. As observed in other studies [59], differences between samples at baseline and at the end of follow-up were much more profound in the RYGB group: the phyla Pseudomonadota, Bacteroidota, Verrucomicrobiota, and Fusobacteriota experienced a significant increase in number at 3 months after RYGB surgery, inversely to Bacillota and Actinomycetota. However, the changes were considerably less marked in the SG group, with a slight enrichment of certain Bacillota, such as *Streptococcus*, *Parvimonas*, *Hungatella*, *Lactobacillus*, and *Desulfovibrio*, along with a decrease in Bacteroidota and Negativicutes. Lastly, and despite these differences in bacterial composition, the authors emphasized that weight loss was uniform in both groups, independent of the initial gut microbiota composition (**Figure 2**).

6.1 Type 2 diabetes mellitus remission

Regarding T2DM remission after BS, discordant results have been published according to a meta-analysis review [60]. This discordance could be explained by the design of the studies, the sample size and statistical power to assess differences, as well as the duration of follow-up. In addition, the authors note that different remission criteria were used in the literature reviewed, which could have possibly led to discrepancies in the interpretation of the available evidence. However, other researchers have explored the possibility that remission of diabetes after RYGB and SG surgery may be associated with interindividual differences in microbiota composition.

Although post-surgical changes in gut microbiota richness and composition were observed, these were independent of T2DM remission status, and no specific postoperative gender signature was identified that discriminated patients who reached this metabolic outcome [59]. However, a distinct genus signature pre-RYGB was observed in patients with total T2DM remission (**Figure 3**).

Murphy et al. [61] found that body weight reduction, dietary changes, and T2DM remission were similar 1 year after both RYGB and SG. RYGB surgery resulted in an

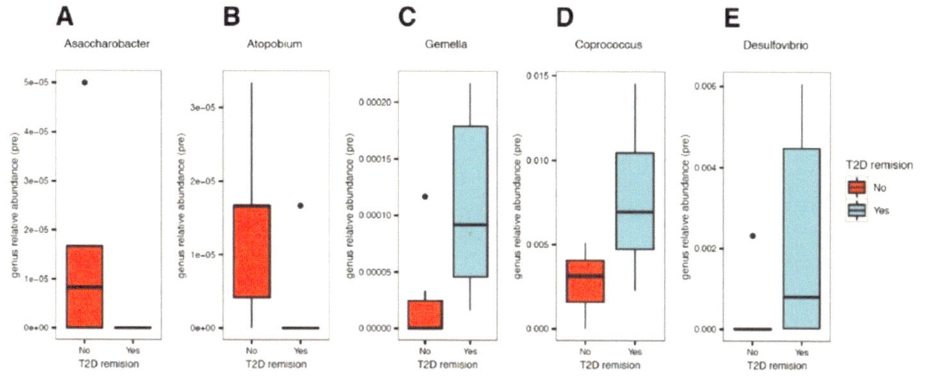

Figure 3.
Gut bacteria genera at the preoperative period in obese patients classified according to T2D remission after RYGB. These figures represent comparison at the preoperative period of gut bacteria genus profile between patients classified, after RYGB, according to presence (blue boxes; n = 8) and absence of T2D remission (red boxes; n = 6). There was a higher relative abundance of (a) Asaccharobacter (p = 0.038) and (B) Atopobium (p = 0.047) and a lower relative abundance of (C) Gemella (p = 0.018), (D) Coprococcus (p = 0.029), and (E) Desulfovibrio (p = 0.030) in the patients with T2D remission than in patients without, (from: Al-Assal K et al. [59]).

increased Bacillota and Actinomycetota phyla, but a decreased Bacteroidota phyla. On the other hand, the SG procedure resulted in an increased Bacteroidota phyla. An increase in *Roseburia* species was observed among those who achieved diabetes remission in both types of surgery, although greater changes in gut microbiota metabolism occurred after RYGB than after SG. Contrary to the findings of Al-Assal et al. [59], those with persistent diabetes postoperatively had more *Desulfovibrio* species before surgery.

Similar results were addressed in Davies et al. [62], a higher abundance of *Eubacteriaceae* and *Alistipes putredinis* was observed before surgery in those individuals with T2DM remission post-intervention. After BS, *Lachnospiraceae* and *Roseburia* species were more abundant in those who had achieved T2DM remission.

The differential bacterial abundance was analyzed in 8 patients who underwent RYGB with complete resolution of diabetes as reported by Salazar et al. in 2022 [58], showing a significant increase of Verrucomicrobiota phyla (*Akkermansia*) and Fusobacteriota (*Fusobacterium*) after surgery, whereas the relative abundance of the phyla Bacillota (*Faecalibacterium*, *Erysipelotrichia*, *Gemmiger*, and *Lactobacillus*) and Actinomycetota (*Bifidobacterium*) decreased.

7. Potential interventions for modulating gut microbiota

There is immense potential for microbiome-modulating therapies based on microbial replacement, which are emerging as a treatment option for several diseases. These new intervention approaches have been made possible by our growing understanding of host-microbiome interactions [63]. Various interventions are possible depending on the level of invasion, ranging from dietary changes to microbial replacement through fecal transplantation (**Figure 4**).

7.1 Diet

As mentioned previously, nutritional recommendations for a Mediterranean diet or plant-based diet, which are rich in polyunsaturated and monounsaturated fat, have

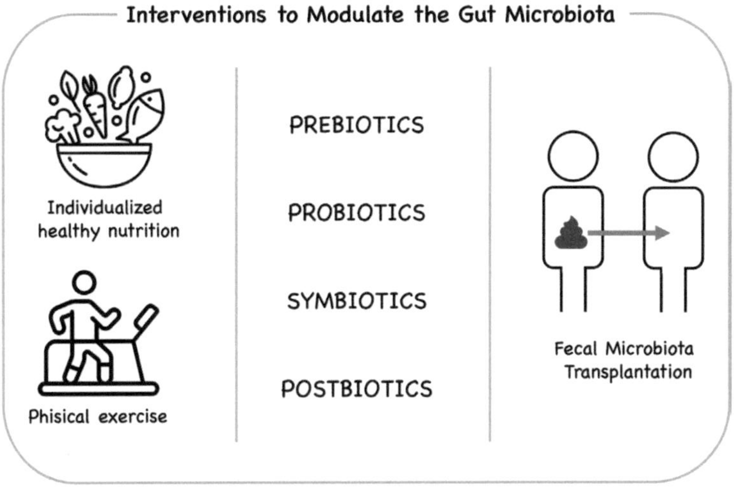

Figure 4.
Different level interventions for gut microbiota modulation.

been associated with higher bacterial diversity, higher levels of total SCFA [64, 65], and significant reductions in plasma cholesterol [66]. Increased physical activity has also demonstrated beneficial changes to the gut microbiome [67]. To establish a clear intervention effect on the gut microbiome through modulation of dietary fat, both in quantity and quality, more clinical trials are needed to establish nutritional recommendations [68].

7.2 The "biotics": Prebiotics, probiotics, symbiotics, and postbiotics

Complex mixtures of bacterial strains (probiotics) and various fiber dosages (prebiotics), which are "symbiotic", have been used in multiple studies regarding obesity treatment. *In vitro* studies have shown that symbiotics are more efficient at modulating gut microbiota than prebiotics or probiotics alone [69].

According to the consensus statement of the International Scientific Association of Probiotics and Prebiotics (ISAPP), postbiotics are defined as "preparations of inanimate microorganisms and/or their components that confer a health benefit on the host" [70]. SCFAs are currently the most common type of postbiotics used. These compounds increase brown adipose tissue and promote browning of white adipose tissue, as well as regulate appetite by interfering with the gut-brain axis [71]. Overall, probiotics, prebiotics, symbiotics, and postbiotics appear to exhibit beneficial effects on gut microbiota modulation. Nevertheless, further large-scale trials are required to evaluate their beneficial properties, safety profile, dosage, and the durability of their beneficial effects in the prevention and treatment of obesity [72].

7.3 Fecal microbiota transplantation (FMT)

FMT is a modulation strategy that transfers a complete microbial ecosystem from a healthy donor to a patient with the aim of ecologically restoring an aberrant microbiota [73]. The donor's microbiota can be administered through colonoscopy or orally by capsules. This technique has been widely investigated for the treatment of recurrent *Clostridioides difficile* infection, with outstanding therapeutic success rates; however, there is no current indication for obesity [74].

Although several studies have been performed in patients with various inflammatory disorders, such as irritable bowel syndrome and obesity-associated metabolic disorders, therapeutic success rates were not as high, or no effect was observed [75–77].

Further studies are required to understand the mechanisms through which changes in gut microbial ecology and engraftment of microbiota affect metabolic outcomes for patients with obesity. In addition, further research is needed to better define the optimal fecal microbial preparation as well as dosing and method of delivery [78].

8. Final conclusions

- Even with valuable insights into the impact of the microbiome on human health and disease, our understanding is limited due to the highly individualized profile of the microbiome and its complex multi-directional interactions with the human host.

- The development of sampling methods is critical for future gut microbiota research, given that the correct sampling has a crucial effect on the accuracy of "omics" techniques.

- Future larger studies using high-throughput sequencing and metagenomic and metabolomic techniques will provide a better understanding of the composition of the microbiota and its functional evolution after BS.

- Although further investigation is required, combining various modulation strategies, such as diet, biotics, and in certain cases, FMT, might be the best approach to "normalize" the gut microbiota as prophylaxis therapy when patients are going under BS.

- The gut microbiota influences several aspects of human health, from innate immunity to energy and metabolism. Modulation of the gut microbiome could therefore potentially reduce obesity and should be based on dietary interventions and lifestyle changes.

Acknowledgements

The authors are grateful to the Bariatric Surgery Unit of the Hospital Ramón y Cajal, and to the patients. we would like to thank all the people who have contributed to this work, especially Marta Cobo and Yolanda Gutiérrez.

This work was supported by the Spanish Ministry of Science and Innovation, Instituto de Salud Carlos III (ICI21/00012), and co-funded by the NextGenerationEU and PRTR. MPA was supported by a Rio Hortega contract (CM19/00069) and JA by a Sara Borrell contract (CD21/00059), both from the Instituto de Salud Carlos III and co-funded by the European Social Fund (ESF, "Investing in your future").

Conflict of interest

The authors declare no conflict of interest.

DOI: http://dx.doi.org/10.5772/intechopen.107175

Author details

Natalia Bastón-Paz[1,2,3*], Manuel Ponce-Alonso[1,2,3], José Avendaño[1,2,3], María Garriga[2,4] and Rosa del Campo[1]

1 Department of Microbiology, University Hospital Ramón y Cajal, Madrid, Spain

2 Instituto Ramón y Cajal de Investigación Sanitaria (IRYCIS), Madrid, Spain

3 CIBERINFEC, Madrid, Spain

4 Department of Endocrinology and Nutrition, University Hospital Ramón y Cajal, Madrid, Spain

*Address all correspondence to: natalia.baston.paz@gmail.com

References

[1] Baquero F, Nombela C. The microbiome as a human organ. Clinical Microbiology and Infection. 2012;**18**(Suppl. 4):2-4. DOI: 10.1111/j.1469-0691.2012.03916.x

[2] Ramirez J, Guarner F, Bustos Fernandez L, Maruy A, Sdepanian VL, Cohen H. Antibiotics as major disruptors of gut microbiota. Frontiers in Cellular and Infection Microbiology. 2020;**10**:572912. DOI: 10.3389/fcimb.2020.572912

[3] Tseng CH, Wu CY. The gut microbiome in obesity. Journal of the Formosan Medical Association. 2019;**118**(Suppl. 1):S3-S9. DOI: 10.1016/j.jfma.2018.07.009

[4] Gomaa EZ. Human gut microbiota/microbiome in health and diseases: A review. Antonie Van Leeuwenhoek. 2020;**113**:2019-2040. DOI: 10.1007/s10482-020-01474-7

[5] Lynch SV, Pedersen O. The human intestinal microbiome in health and disease. The New England Journal of Medicine. 2016;**375**:2369-2379. DOI: 10.1056/NEJMra1600266

[6] Lau JT, Whelan FJ, Herath I, Lee CH, Collins SM, Bercik P, et al. Capturing the diversity of the human gut microbiota through culture-enriched molecular profiling. Genome Medicine. 2016;**8**:72. DOI: 10.1186/s13073-016-0327-7

[7] Lagier JC, Dubourg G, Million M, Cadoret F, Bilen M, Fenollar F, et al. Culturing the human microbiota and culturomics. Nature Reviews. Microbiology. 2018;**16**:540-550. DOI: 10.1038/s41579-018-0041-0

[8] Berg G, Rybakova D, Fischer D, Cernava T, Vergès MC, Charles T, et al. Microbiome definition re-visited: Old concepts and new challenges. Microbiome. 2020;**8**:103. DOI: 10.1186/s40168-020-00875-0

[9] Pérez-Cobas AE, Gomez-Valero L, Buchrieser C. Metagenomic approaches in microbial ecology: An update on whole-genome and marker gene sequencing analyses. Microbial Genomics. 2020;**6**:mgen000409. DOI: 10.1099/mgen.0.000409

[10] Vaga S, Lee S, Ji B, Andreasson A, Talley NJ, Agréus L, et al. Compositional and functional differences of the mucosal microbiota along the intestine of healthy individuals. Scientific Reports. 2020;**10**:14977. DOI: 10.1038/s41598-020-71939-2

[11] Kim D, Jung JY, Oh HS, Jee SR, Park SJ, Lee SH, et al. Comparison of sampling methods in assessing the microbiome from patients with ulcerative colitis. BMC Gastroenterology. 2021;**21**:396. DOI: 10.1186/s12876-021-01975-3

[12] Tang Q, Jin G, Wang G, Liu T, Liu X, Wang B, et al. Current sampling methods for gut microbiota: A call for more precise devices. Frontiers in Cellular and Infection Microbiology. 2020;**10**:151. DOI: 10.3389/fcimb.2020.00151

[13] Hill C, Ross RP, Stanton C, O'Toole PW. The human microbiome in health and disease. In: Unden G, Thines E, Schüffler A, editors. Host – Pathogen Interaction. Wiley-VCH Verlag GmBH &Co. KgaA; 2016. DOI: 10.1002/9783527682386.ch4

[14] Finotello F, Mastrorilli E, Di Camillo B. Measuring the diversity of the human microbiota with targeted

next-generation sequencing. Briefings in Bioinformatics. 2018;**19**:679-692. DOI: 10.1093/bib/bbw119

[15] Walters KE, Martiny JBH. Alpha-, beta-, and gamma-diversity of bacteria varies across habitats. PLoS One. 2020;**15**:e0233872. DOI: 10.1371/journal.pone.0233872

[16] Ponce-Alonso M, García-Fernández S, del Campo R. Challenges of landscaping and modulation strategies in human intestinal microbiota. Enfermedades Infecciosas y Microbiologia Clinica. 2021;**39**:165-167. DOI: 10.1016/j.cimc.2021.02.001

[17] Fan Y, Pedersen O. Gut microbiota in human metabolic health and disease. Nature Reviews. Microbiology. 2021;**19**:55-71. DOI: 10.1038/s41579-020-0433-9

[18] Mousa WK, Chehadeh F, Husband S. Recent advances in understanding the structure and function of the human microbiome. Frontiers in Microbiology. 2022;**13**:825338. DOI: 10.3389/fmicb.2022.825338

[19] Moore RE, Townsend SD. Temporal development of the infant gut microbiome. Open Biology. 2019;**9**:190128. DOI: 10.1098/rsob.190128

[20] Tamburini S, Shen N, Wu HC, Clemente JC. The microbiome in early life: Implications for health outcomes. Nature Medicine. 2016;**22**:713-722. DOI: 10.1038/nm.4142

[21] Kim H, Sitarik AR, Woodcroft K, Johnson CC, Zoratti E. Birth mode, breastfeeding, pet exposure, and antibiotic use: Associations with the gut microbiome and sensitization in children. Current Allergy and Asthma Reports. 2019;**19**:22. DOI: 10.1007/s11882-019-0851-9

[22] Davis EC, Wang M, Donovan SM. The role of early life nutrition in the establishment of gastrointestinal microbial composition and function. Gut Microbes. 2017;**8**:143-171. DOI: 10.1080/19490976.2016.1278104

[23] Panda S, El khader I, Casellas F, López Vivancos J, García Cors M, Santiago A, et al. Short-term effect of antibiotics on human gut microbiota. PLoS One. 2014;**9**:e95476. DOI: 10.1371/journal.pone.0095476

[24] Escudero-Sánchez R, Ponce-Alonso M, Barragán-Prada H, Morosini MI, Cantón R, Cobo J, et al. Long-term impact of suppressive antibiotic therapy on intestinal microbiota. Genes (Basel). 2020;**12**:41. DOI: 10.3390/genes12010041

[25] Konstantinidis T, Tsigalou C, Karvelas A, Stavropoulou E, Voidarou C, Bezirtzoglou E. Effects of antibiotics upon the gut microbiome: A review of the literature. Biomedicine. 2020;**8**:502. DOI: 10.3390/biomedicines8110502

[26] Cox LM, Blaser MJ. Antibiotics in early life and obesity. Nature Reviews. Endocrinology. 2015;**11**:182-190. DOI: 10.1038/nrendo.2014.210

[27] Garcia-Mantrana I, Selma-Royo M, Alcantara C, Collado MC. Shifts on gut microbiota associated to mediterranean diet adherence and specific dietary intakes on general adult population. Frontiers in Microbiology. 2018;**9**:890. DOI: 10.3389/fmicb.2018.00890

[28] Kim CH, Park J, Kim M. Gut microbiota-derived short-chain fatty acids, T cells, and inflammation. Immune Network. 2014;**14**:277-288. DOI: 10.4110/in.2014.14.6.277

[29] Graf D, Di Cagno R, Fåk F, Flint HJ, Nyman M, Saarela M, et al. Contribution

of diet to the composition of the human gut microbiota. Microbial Ecology in Health and Disease. 2015;**26**:26164. DOI: 10.3402/mehd.v26.26164

[30] Bressa C, Bailén-Andrino M, Pérez-Santiago J, González-Soltero R, Pérez M, Montalvo-Lominchar MG, et al. Differences in gut microbiota profile between women with active lifestyle and sedentary women. PLoS One. 2017;**12**:e0171352. DOI: 10.1371/journal.pone.0171352

[31] Fouladi F, Bailey MJ, Patterson WB, Sioda M, Blakley IC, Fodor AA, et al. Air pollution exposure is associated with the gut microbiome as revealed by shotgun metagenomic sequencing. Environment International. 2020;**138**:105604. DOI: 10.1016/j.envint.2020.105604

[32] Lee SH, Yun Y, Kim SJ, Lee EJ, Chang Y, Ryu S, et al. Association between cigarette smoking status and composition of gut microbiota: Population-based cross-sectional study. Journal of Clinical Medicine. 2018;**7**:282. DOI: 10.3390/jcm7090282

[33] Zhang D, Li S, Wang N, Tan HY, Zhang Z, Feng Y. The cross-talk between gut microbiota and lungs in common lung diseases. Frontiers in Microbiology. 2020;**11**:301. DOI: 10.3389/fmicb.2020.00301

[34] Suganya K, Koo BS. Gut-brain Axis: Role of gut microbiota on neurological disorders and how probiotics/prebiotics beneficially modulate microbial and immune pathways to improve brain functions. International Journal of Molecular Sciences. 2020;**21**:7551. DOI: 10.3390/ijms21207551

[35] Rosshart SP, Herz J, Vassallo BG, Hunter A, Wall MK, Badger JH, et al. Laboratory mice born to wild mice have natural microbiota and model human immune responses. Science. 2019;**365**:eaaw4361. DOI: 10.1126/science.aaw4361

[36] Sjögren K, Engdahl C, Henning P, Lerner UH, Tremaroli V, Lagerquist MK, et al. The gut microbiota regulates bone mass in mice. Journal of Bone and Mineral Research. 2012;**27**:1357-1367. DOI: 10.1002/jbmr.1588

[37] Ohlsson C, Nigro G, Boneca IG, Bäckhed F, Sansonetti P, Sjögren K. Regulation of bone mass by the gut microbiota is dependent on NOD1 and NOD2 signaling. Cellular Immunology. 2017;**317**:55-58. DOI: 10.1016/j.cellimm.2017.05.003

[38] Rackaityte E, Lynch SV. The human microbiome in the 21st century. Nature Communications. 2020;**11**:5256. DOI: 10.1038/s41467-020-18983-8

[39] He W, Luo Y, Liu JP, Sun N, Guo D, Cui LL, et al. Trimethylamine N-oxide, a gut microbiota-dependent metabolite, is associated with frailty in older adults with cardiovascular disease. Clinical Interventions in Aging. 2020;**15**:1809-1820. DOI: 10.2147/CIA.S270887

[40] Wharton S, Lau DCW, Vallis M, Sharma AM, Biertho L, Campbell-Scherer D, et al. Obesity in adults: A clinical practice guideline. CMAJ. 2020;**192**:E875-E891. DOI: 10.1503/cmaj.191707

[41] Turnbaugh PJ, Ley RE, Mahowald MA, Magrini V, Mardis ER, Gordon JI. An obesity-associated gut microbiome with increased capacity for energy harvest. Nature. 2006;**444**:1027-1031. DOI: 10.1038/nature05414

[42] Bervoets L, Van Hoorenbeeck K, Kortleven I, Van Noten C, Hens N, Vael C, et al. Differences in gut microbiota composition between obese and

lean children: A cross-sectional study. Gut Pathogens. 2013;**5**:10. DOI: 10.1186/1757-4749-5-10

[43] Campisciano G, Palmisano S, Cason C, Giuricin M, Silvestri M, Guerra M, et al. Gut microbiota characterisation in obese patients before and after bariatric surgery. Beneficial Microbes. 2018;**9**:367-373. DOI: 10.3920/BM2017.0152

[44] Magne F, Gotteland M, Gauthier L, Zazueta A, Pesoa S, Navarrete P, et al. The Firmicutes/Bacteroidetes ratio: A relevant marker of gut dysbiosis in obese patients? Nutrients. 2020 May;**12**:1474. DOI: 10.3390/nu12051474

[45] Pinart M, Dötsch A, Schlicht K, Laudes M, Bouwman J, Forslund SK, et al. Gut microbiome composition in obese and non-obese persons: A systematic review and meta-analysis. Nutrients. 2021;**14**:12. DOI: 10.3390/nu14010012

[46] Crovesy L, Masterson D, Rosado EL. Profile of the gut microbiota of adults with obesity: A systematic review. European Journal of Clinical Nutrition. 2020;**74**:1251-1262. DOI: 10.1038/s41430-020-0607-6

[47] Allin KH, Tremaroli V, Caesar R, Jensen BAH, Damgaard MTF, Bahl MI, et al. Aberrant intestinal microbiota in individuals with prediabetes. Diabetologia. 2018;**61**:810-820. DOI: 10.1007/s00125-018-4550-1

[48] Zhong H, Ren H, Lu Y, Fang C, Hou G, Yang Z, et al. Distinct gut metagenomics and metaproteomics signatures in prediabetics and treatment-naïve type 2 diabetics. eBioMedicine. 2019;**47**:373-383. DOI: 10.1016/j.ebiom.2019.08.048

[49] de la Cuesta-Zuluaga J, Mueller NT, Corrales-Agudelo V, Velásquez-Mejía EP, Carmona JA, Abad JM, et al. Metformin is associated with higher relative abundance of mucin-degrading *Akkermansia muciniphila* and several short-chain fatty acid-producing microbiota in the gut. Diabetes Care. 2017;**40**:54-62. DOI: 10.2337/dc16-1324

[50] Bryrup T, Thomsen CW, Kern T, Allin KH, Brandslund I, Jørgensen NR, et al. Metformin-induced changes of the gut microbiota in healthy young men: Results of a non-blinded, one-armed intervention study. Diabetologia. 2019;**62**:1024-1035. DOI: 10.1007/s00125-019-4848-7

[51] Vallianou NG, Stratigou T, Tsagarakis S. Metformin and gut microbiota: Their interactions and their impact on diabetes. Hormones (Athens, Greece). 2019;**18**:141-144. DOI: 10.1007/s42000-019-00093-w

[52] Wharton S, Lau DCW, Vallis M, et al. Obesity in adults: A clinical practice guideline. CMAJ. 2020;**192**:E875-E891. DOI: 10.1503/cmaj.191707

[53] Magouliotis DE, Tasiopoulou VS, Sioka E, Chatedaki C, Zacharoulis D. Impact of bariatric surgery on metabolic and gut microbiota profile: A systematic review and meta-analysis. Obesity Surgery. 2017;**27**:1345-1357. DOI: 10.1007/s11695-017-2595-8

[54] Mika A, Janczy A, Waleron K, Szymanski M, Kaska L, Sledzinski T. The impact of the interplay of the intestinal microbiome and diet on the metabolomic and health outcomes of bariatric surgery. Obesity Reviews. 2022;**8**:e13455. DOI: 10.1111/obr.13455

[55] Aron-Wisnewsky J, Doré J, Clement K. The importance of the gut microbiota after bariatric surgery. Nature Reviews. Gastroenterology & Hepatology. 2012;**9**:590-598. DOI: 10.1038/nrgastro.2012.161

[56] Oduro-Donkor D, Turner MC, Farnaud S, Renshaw D, Kyrou I, Hanson P, et al. Modification of fecal microbiota as a mediator of effective weight loss and metabolic benefits following bariatric surgery. Expert Review of Endocrinology and Metabolism. 2020;**15**:363-373. DOI: 10.1080/17446651.2020.1801412

[57] Juárez-Fernández M, Román-Sagüillo S, Porras D, García-Mediavilla MV, Linares P, Ballesteros-Pomar MD, et al. Long-term effects of bariatric surgery on gut microbiota composition and faecal metabolome related to obesity remission. Nutrients. 2021;**13**:2519. DOI: 10.3390/nu13082519

[58] Salazar N, Ponce-Alonso M, Garriga M, et al. Fecal metabolome and bacterial composition in severe obesity: Impact of diet and bariatric surgery. Research Square. Gut Microbes. 2022;**14**:2106102. DOI: 10.1080/19490976.2022.2106102

[59] Al Assal K, Prifti E, Belda E, Sala P, Clément K, Dao MC, et al. Gut microbiota profile of obese diabetic women submitted to roux-en-Y gastric bypass and its association with food intake and postoperative diabetes remission. Nutrients. 2020;**12**:278. DOI: 10.3390/nu12020278 PMID: 31973130

[60] Castellana M, Procino F, Biacchi E, Zupo R, Lampignano L, Castellana F, et al. Roux-en-Y gastric bypass vs sleeve gastrectomy for remission of type 2 diabetes. The Journal of Clinical Endocrinology and Metabolism. 2021;**106**:922-933. DOI: 10.1210/clinem/dgaa737

[61] Murphy R, Tsai P, Jüllig M, Liu A, Plank L, Booth M. Differential changes in gut microbiota after gastric bypass and sleeve gastrectomy bariatric surgery vary according to diabetes remission. Obesity Surgery. 2017;**27**:917-925. DOI: 10.1007/s11695-016-2399-2

[62] Davies N, O'Sullivan JM, Plank LD, Murphy R. Gut microbial predictors of type 2 diabetes remission following bariatric surgery. Obesity Surgery. 2020;**30**:3536-3548. DOI: 10.1007/s11695-020-04684-0

[63] Gupta A, Saha S, Khanna S. Therapies to modulate gut microbiota: Past, present and future. World Journal of Gastroenterology. 2020;**26**:777-788. DOI: 10.3748/wjg.v26.i8.777

[64] Garcia-Mantrana I, Selma-Royo M, Alcantara C, Collado MC. Shifts on gut microbiota associated to mediterranean diet adherence and specific dietary intakes on general adult population. Frontiers in Microbiology. 2018;**9**:890. DOI: 10.3389/fmicb.2018.00890

[65] Muralidharan J, Galiè S, Hernández-Alonso P, Bulló M, Salas-Salvadó J. Plant-based fat, dietary patterns rich in vegetable fat and gut microbiota modulation. Frontiers in Nutrition. 2019 Oct;**6**:157. DOI: 10.3389/fnut.2019.00157

[66] Meslier V, Laiola M, Roager HM, De Filippis F, Roume H, Quinquis B, et al. Mediterranean diet intervention in overweight and obese subjects lowers plasma cholesterol and causes changes in the gut microbiome and metabolome independently of energy intake. Gut. 2020;**69**:1258-1268. DOI: 10.1136/gutjnl-2019-320438

[67] Monda V, Villano I, Messina A, Valenzano A, Esposito T, Moscatelli F, et al. Exercise modifies the gut microbiota with positive health effects. Oxidative Medicine and Cellular Longevity. 2017;**2017**:3831972. DOI: 10.1155/2017/3831972

[68] Wolters M, Ahrens J, Romaní-Pérez M, Watkins C, Sanz Y, Benítez-Páez A, et al. Dietary fat, the gut microbiota, and metabolic health - a systematic review conducted within the MyNewGut project. Clinical Nutrition. 2019;**38**:2504-2520. DOI: 10.1016/j.clnu.2018.12.024

[69] Krumbeck JA, Rasmussen HE, Hutkins RW, Clarke J, Shawron K, Keshavarzian A, et al. Probiotic *Bifidobacterium* strains and galactooligosaccharides improve intestinal barrier function in obese adults but show no synergism when used together as synbiotics. Microbiome. 2018;**6**:121. DOI: 10.1186/s40168-018-0494-4

[70] Salminen S, Collado MC, Endo A, Hill C, Lebeer S, Quigley EMM, et al. The international scientific Association of Probiotics and Prebiotics (ISAPP) consensus statement on the definition and scope of postbiotics. Nature Reviews. Gastroenterology & Hepatology. 2021;**18**:649-667. DOI: 10.1038/s41575-021-00440-6

[71] Żółkiewicz J, Marzec A, Ruszczyński M, Feleszko W. Postbiotics-a step beyond pre- and probiotics. Nutrients. 2020;**12**:2189. DOI: 10.3390/nu12082189

[72] Vallianou N, Stratigou T, Christodoulatos GS, Tsigalou C, Dalamaga M. Probiotics, prebiotics, synbiotics, postbiotics, and obesity: Current evidence, controversies, and perspectives. Current Obesity Reports. 2020;**9**:179-192. DOI: 10.1007/s13679-020-00379-w

[73] Falony G, Vandeputte D, Caenepeel C, Vieira-Silva S, Daryoush T, Vermeire S, et al. The human microbiome in health and disease: Hype or hope. Acta Clinica Belgica. 2019;**74**:53-64. DOI: 10.1080/17843286.2019.1583782

[74] Cammarota G, Ianiro G, Tilg H, Rajilić-Stojanović M, Kump P, Satokari R, et al. European FMT working group. European consensus conference on faecal microbiota transplantation in clinical practice. Gut. 2017;**66**:569-580. DOI: 10.1136/gutjnl-2016-313017

[75] Colman RJ, Rubin DT. Fecal microbiota transplantation as therapy for inflammatory bowel disease: A systematic review and meta-analysis. Journal of Crohn's & Colitis. 2014;**8**:1569-1581. DOI: 10.1016/j.crohns.2014.08.006

[76] Halkjær SI, Christensen AH, Lo BZS, Browne PD, Günther S, Hansen LH, et al. Faecal microbiota transplantation alters gut microbiota in patients with irritable bowel syndrome: Results from a randomised, double-blind placebo-controlled study. Gut. 2018;**67**:2107-2115. DOI: 10.1136/gutjnl-2018-316434

[77] Leong KSW, Jayasinghe TN, Wilson BC, Derraik JGB, Albert BB, Chiavaroli V, et al. Effects of fecal microbiome transfer in adolescents with obesity: The gut bugs randomized controlled trial. JAMA Network Open. 2020;**3**:e2030415. DOI: 10.1001/jamanetworkopen.2020.30415

[78] Zhang Z, Mocanu V, Cai C, Dang J, Slater L, Deehan EC, et al. Impact of fecal microbiota transplantation on obesity and metabolic syndrome-a systematic review. Nutrients. 2019;**11**:2291. DOI: 10.3390/nu11102291

Chapter 8

Outcomes of Bariatric Surgery

Asad Ullah

Abstract

The prevalence of obesity has increased globally. Management of obesity consists of medical and surgical interventions. The results of bariatric surgery are consistently more significant than medical therapy. Importantly, bariatric surgery achieves durable weight loss in more patients than medical therapy. Moreover, studies have reported improvement in most obesity-related complications after bariatric surgery. Improvement or remission of type 2 diabetes mellitus, hypertension and dyslipidemia is noteworthy. Due to better outcomes, the indications of bariatric surgery are expanding. In conclusion, bariatric surgery is a cost-effective and safer alternative for morbidly obese patients who fail to respond to non-surgical treatments. Some studies have raised concerns about the worsening of mental health problems after bariatric surgerys. It requires careful management of high-risk patients and further research.

Keywords: obesity, bariatric surgery, weight loss, metabolic and other outcomes

1. Introduction

The global prevalence of obesity has tripled since 1975 [1]. Obesity is managed according to the severity and associated comorbid conditions. Bariatric surgery is recommended for class II obesity with associated comorbidities and class III obesity. It confers the most effective and durable weight loss. The number of bariatric procedures in the United States has significantly increased in the last decade [2].

The primary outcome of bariatric surgery is weight loss; however, it also improves obesity-related comorbidities and overall survival.

Bariatric surgery has progressed significantly since its origin in 1954. In contemporary practice, Roux-en-Y gastric bypass surgery (RYGB), sleeve gastrectomy (SG) and adjustable gastric band (AGB) are the most performed procedures. This chapter will focus on the outcomes of these three surgical techniques.

2. Outcomes of bariatric surgery

2.1 Weight loss

Weight loss is the primary goal of bariatric surgery. Regardless of the procedure, bariatric surgery provides significant long-term weight loss compared to non-surgical therapies [3].

There is no standardized metric for reporting weight loss. In surgical literature, it is frequently reported as the percentage of excess weight loss (EWL) as shown in Eq. (1) [4]

$$\%EWL = (\text{Pre bariatric surgery (BS) weight} - \text{Post BS weight}) / (\text{Pre BS weight} - \text{ideal body weight}) * 100 \quad (1)$$

Ideal body weight is conventionally determined by using Metropolitan Life Tables [5] or the method of the Devine [6].

Some authors used percentage excess body mass index (BMI) loss (as shown in Eq. (2)) [4],

$$\%BMIL = (\text{Pre BS BMI} - \text{Post BS BMI}) / (\text{Pre BS BMI} - 25) * 100 \quad (2)$$

In the medical literature, weight loss is reported as a percentage of total weight loss (TWL) expressed as Eq. (3) [4],

$$\%TWL = (\text{Pre BS weight} - \text{Post BS weight}) / \text{Pre BS weight} * 100 \quad (3)$$

These parameters have limitations; however, %TWL is most frequently reported in contemporary literature.

Weight loss post-bariatric surgery is highly variable. Initially, a rapid weight decline is observed in the first 6 months, reaching a peak at 12 months. Then it slows down and reaches a plateau between 1 and 1.5 years (see **Table 1**).

Weight loss after RYGB & SG is comparable. Swiss multicenter bypass or sleeve study (SM-BOSS) [8] reported similar weight loss after RYGB and SG at 2, 3 and 5 years. Improvements in metabolic outcomes such as remission of diabetes mellitus (DM), hypertension (HTN) and hyperlipidemia were also comparable.

Laparoscopic Sleeve Gastrectomy vs. laparoscopic Roux en Y gastric bypass (SLEEVEPASS) study [9] showed greater excess weight loss with RYGB compared to SG (55 vs. 47% at 7 years).

Observational studies illustrate higher weight loss with RYGB than SG [10, 11]. It is likely related to the study design.

Weight loss with AGB is slower, reaching a plateau at 2 years [7]. The longitudinal assessment of bariatric surgery (LABS) study [12] compared RYGB and laparoscopic AGB in a cohort of 2348 obese individuals. At seven years, the mean weight loss with

Surgical technique	% Excess weight loss	Time for weight stabilization (year)
AGB	45–55	2
SG	55–80	1–1.5
RYGB	60–85	1–1.5

Table 1.
Expected weight loss after bariatric surgery [7].

RYGB was 38.2 kg (95% CI, 36.9–39.5) and 18.8 kg (95% CI 16.3–21.3) after AGB. Due to lack of efficacy, the reoperation rate was higher in the AGB group than in the RYGB group (n = 160 vs. 14).

Adjustable gastric banding has gone out of practice due to lack of efficacy.

Most of the patients will regain some weight regardless of the operation commencing in the second year. It is estimated to be 5–10% of TBW in the first 10 years; e.g., in the Swedish obese subjects (SOS) study, the TWL decreased from 32 to 25% at 10 years after RYGB [13]. Similarly, in the LABS study, TWL decreased from 35 to 28% after RYGB [12].

What is the significant weight regain is not clearly defined in the literature. The risk of weight regain is lowest for RYGB (2.5 to 3.3%), followed by SG (12.5 to 14.5%) and highest for AGB (30.5 to 36%) [10, 14].

2.2 Metabolic benefits

Metabolic syndrome or insulin resistance is the co-existence of risk factors for cardiovascular diseases and type 2 diabetes mellitus (T2DM) including hypertension, central obesity, high blood glucose level and dyslipidemia. Bariatric surgery is by far the most effective treatment for metabolic syndrome. The effects of bariatric surgery on each component of metabolic syndrome are discussed below.

2.2.1 Effects on type 2 diabetes mellitus

Durable remission of T2DM is reported in 23 to 60% of cases [15]. Glycemic control improves within days after the surgery suggesting the role of weight loss independent factors. Bariatric surgery influences β-cell function, incretin responses, insulin sensitivity, gut microbiota, bile composition, intestinal glucose metabolism and brown adipose tissue metabolism [16, 17]. Weight loss contributes to better glycemic control in the long run. A French national survey study demonstrated the preventative role of bariatric surgery in T2DM [18]. The risk of developing T2DM was lower in the surgery group than medical therapy group [2 vs. 13% hazard ratio (H.R.) 0.18, 95% CI: 0.17–0.19]. Roux en Y gastric bypass and SG conferred better protection against T2DM than AGB (1.2 vs. 0.9 vs. 4.5%, respectively). Patients with a shorter duration of T2DM, better pre-operation glycemic control and significant weight loss post-surgery had higher chances of achieving remission.

Many prospective and retrospective studies have shown favorable effects of bariatric surgery on the management of T2DM. A meta-analysis [19] reported higher rates of T2DM remission with RYGB than medical therapy at 1 year [RR, 18.01; 95% CI: 4.53–71.70], 3 years (RR, 29.58; 95% CI: 5.92–147.82) and 5 years (RR, 16.92; 95% CI: 4.15–69.00). Moreover, a higher proportion of patients in the RYGB group achieved the American Diabetes Association (ADA) treatment targets at 1, 2, 3 & 5 yr.

Another meta-analysis [20] comprising mainly of observational studies reported a T2DM remission rate of 78% and an improvement rate of 87% at 1–3 years follow-up.

A prospective multi-center study [21] compared SG to RYGB and AGB. Type 2 diabetes mellitus improved or remitted in 83, 55 and 44% with RYGB, SG & AGB respectively at 1 year.

Most observational studies show better remission rates of T2DM with RYGB than SG. However, prospective studies demonstrate comparable efficacy of RYGB and SG inducing T2DM remission [8, 22]. The effectiveness of AGB is low in this regard.

Remission of T2DM induced by bariatric surgery is more durable than medical management. A French population-based cohort study illustrated that a greater proportion of patients in the surgery group (RYGB, SG & AGB) were able to discontinue antidiabetic medications at 6 years than medical therapy alone (−49.9% vs. −9.0%, $P < .001$) [23]. Roux-en-Y gastric bypass surgery was more effective in discontinuation of antidiabetic medication than SG and AGB.

A single center study [24] randomly assigned 150 obese participants with uncontrolled T2DM were assigned to either intensive medical therapy alone or medical therapy + RYGB or SG. The primary endpoint was lowering HbA1c to <6% at 12 months. More patients in RYGB and SG groups achieved the primary endpoint than medical therapy alone (42, 37 and 12%, respectively).

Another study randomly assigned obese patients with poorly controlled T2DM to medical therapy alone or RYGB or biliary pancreatic diversion (BPD) [25]. The primary aim was remission of T2DM (fasting blood glucose <5.6 mmol/l and HbA1c < 6.5% without medication) was achieved by 0, 75 and 95% of participants with medical therapy alone, RYGB and BPD, respectively. Type 2 diabetes mellitus remained in remission at 10 years in 5.5, 25 and 50% with medical treatment alone, RYGB and BPD, respectively.

2.2.2 Effects on diabetic mellitus complications

Several retrospective studies illustrate the beneficial effects of bariatric surgery on macrovascular and microvascular complications of T2DM.

A retrospective study reported lower composite macrovascular events in the surgery group than in the medical therapy group [2.1 vs. 4.3%, HR 0.60 (95% CI: 0.42–0.86)] at median 5 years follow-up [26].

Another large retrospective study [27] looked at the extended major adverse cardiovascular event (MACE) in diabetic obese individuals who underwent bariatric surgery or medical therapy. At 8 years, the cumulative incidence of MACE was 30.8% (95% CI: 27.6%–34.0%) in the surgical group vs. 47.7% (95% CI: 46.1%–49.2%) in medical treatment group.

A meta-analysis [28] of 19 studies concluded lower mortality [OR 0.34; 95% CI: (0.25–0.46)] and T2DM macrovascular complications [OR 0.38, (95% CI: 0.22–0.67)] with bariatric surgery compared to medical treatment.

A large cohort study [29] reported a lower incidence of microvascular complications in patients who had bariatric surgery than medical treatment at a median follow-up of 4.3 years [16.9 vs. 34.7% HR 0.41 (95% CI: 0.29–0.58)]. Diabetic neuropathy improved the most among microvascular complications [7.2 vs. 21.4% HR, 0.37 (95% CI: 0.30–0.47)].

In summary, bariatric surgery plus medical therapy induces sustainable remission of T2DM in a significant proportion of patients than medical therapy alone. Bariatric surgery also has favorable effects on the complications of T2DM. Remission of T2DM has a 'legacy effect' or 'metabolic memory' [30], which protects against microvascular complications even after relapse of T2DM.

Most of the guidelines recommend bariatric surgery for patients with class III obesity (BMI $\geq$ 40 kg/m^2) or class II obesity (BMI 35–39.9 kg/m^2) with significant comorbidities. However, clinicians have a growing consensus to consider bariatric surgery for uncontrolled T2DM with medical therapy even with less severe obesity. Bariatric surgery with the primary intent to treat the metabolic syndrome of T2DM is called metabolic surgery. The Diabetes Surgery Summit

(DSS-II) consensus conference guidelines [31] recommend metabolic surgery for patients with poorly controlled T2DM with oral or injectable treatments and class I obesity [BMI 30–34.9 kg/m^2 (27.5–32.4 kg/m^2 for the Asian population)]. DSS-II recommendations are endorsed by American Diabetes Association and many other organizations [32].

2.2.3 Hypertension (HTN)

Hypertension improves with weight loss. The role of bariatric surgery in managing HTN was best demonstrated by the Gastric bypass to treat obese patients with steady hypertension (GATWAY) trial [33]. The study population randomly received medical therapy alone or RYGB + medical therapy. The primary aim was to reduce antihypertensives by ≥30% compared to baseline. More patients in RYGB + medical therapy group achieved the primary endpoint than medical therapy alone at 1 year (84 vs. 13%) and 5 years (73 vs. 11%). A significant proportion of patients in the RYGB group achieved remission of HTN at 1 (46 to 0%) and 5 years (31 to 2%) compared to medical therapy. Moreover, variability in ambulatory blood pressure was low in the RYGB group compared to medical treatment.

A Norwegian cohort study reported HTN remission in 31.9% of individuals who underwent bariatric surgery + medical therapy versus 12.4% in the medical treatment alone group at 6.5 years [34].

What surgical procedure is more efficacious in inducing HTN remission is not clear [21, 35].

2.2.4 Dyslipidemia

Dyslipidemia improves with weight loss. Two meta-analyses showed improvement in serum lipids after bariatric surgery in the short term (< 3 years) [36, 37]. Studies with longer follow-up are required.

A multi-center observational study reported improvement in serum lipids with RYGB compared to baseline (14 vs. 33% for high low-density lipoprotein (LDL) cholesterol; 5 vs. 24% for high triglycerides (TG); 6 vs. 35% for low high-density lipoprotein (HDL) cholesterol) at 7 years. Other observational studies illustrated similar results [38, 39].

2.3 Risk of cancer

Obesity increases the risk of certain cancers such as colon, breast, endometrial, pancreatic, prostate and renal cancers [40, 41]. The outcomes of some malignancies are worse in obese individuals [42].

A database study [43] reported a lower incidence of hormone-related cancers in those who had bariatric surgery (OR 0·23, 95% CI: 0·18–0·30). Roux-en-Y gastric bypass surgery resulted in a higher reduction in hormone-related cancers than SG & AGB. However, the risk of colorectal cancer was higher (OR 2·63, 95% CI: 1·17–5·95) in the RYGB group. Other studies did not report this finding consistently [44]. Another database study showed a 34% higher risk of rectal cancer in obese individuals compared to the general population. The risk of colorectal cancer in obese individuals after bariatric surgery was like the general population [45].

Bariatric surgery has favorable effects on the incidence of all skin cancers (adjusted sub-hazard ratio 0.59, 95% CI: 0.35–0.99) [46].

2.4 Long-term survival

Studies have shown improved all-cause mortality in obese individuals who underwent bariatric surgery; however, it remains higher than in the general population.

A prospective study looked at life expectancy in over 5000 patients from the SOS study cohort [47]. After a median follow-up of 20 years, the hazards for deaths due to cardiovascular disease was 0.70 (95% CI: 0.57–0.85), death from cancer was 0.77 (95% CI: 0.61–0.96) and all-cause mortality was 0.77 (95% CI: 0.68–0.87). The median life expectancy was 3.0 years (95% CI: 1.8–4.2) longer in the bariatric surgery group than in controls but 5.5 years shorter than the general population.

Another large observational cohort study reported lower all-cause mortality rate in bariatric surgery group than control group 0.68 (95% CI: 0.57–0.81) [48] at 4.9 yr. Cardiovascular 0.53 (95% CI: 0.34–0.84) and cancer morality 0.54 (95% CI: 0.36–0.80) were also lower in bariatric surgery group.

Another case-control study reported 40% lower adjusted all-cause mortality in a case-control study (37.6 versus 57.1 deaths per 10,000 person-years $p < 0.001$) at 7 years [49]. However, interestingly the rate of deaths due to suicide and accidents were higher in the RYGB group compared to the control group (11.1 versus 6.4 per 10,000 person-years, $p = 0.04$).

2.5 Functional outcomes.

2.5.1 Obstructive sleep apnea (OSA)

Weight loss improves OSA. An RCT explored the role of RYGB and usual medical care on OSA in grade 1 & 2 obesity [50]. At 3-year follow-up, the apnea-hypoxia index (AHI) was reduced to −13.2 in the RYGB group and increased by +5 events/h in the usual care group. The risk of persistent moderate and severe OSA was also lower in the RYGB group.

A meta-analysis reported comparable improvement or remission rate in OSA with RYGB, AGB & SG (79 vs. 77 vs. 86% for, respectively) [51].

Contrary to the above findings, a meta-analysis demonstrated persistent OSA in patients after bariatric surgery despite improvement in AHI score [52]. It is possibly due to a lack of uniformity in respiratory events scoring in the studies. Detailed assessment for OSA is recommended before discontinuing continuous positive pressure airway therapy.

2.5.2 Gastroesophageal reflux disease (GERD)

Gastroesophageal reflux disease is prevalent in the obese population [53]. The influence of bariatric surgery on GERD is variable and depends on the technique.

Gastroesophageal reflux disease improved or remitted in 70% of cases at 1-year follow-up after RYGB [21]. Another prospective study investigated the role of RYGB on pre-existing GERD [54]. At 6 months follow-up, the risk of GERD was lower than before surgery (33 versus 64%). The use of anti-reflux medications and total acid exposure also decreased. De novo reflux symptoms occurred in 10% of the cases.

The effect of SG on GERD is not clear. A retrospective study [55] of the Bariatric longitudinal database (BOLD) showed that GERD symptoms persisted in 84% of the individuals after SG. De novo GERD symptoms manifested in 8.6% of cases. Fifty per cent of patients with pre-existing GERD reported remission or improvement of GERD in another database study [21]. A systematic review [56] reported a lack of consensus in the studies. Gastroesophageal reflux disease and Barrett's esophagus are not absolute contraindications for SG; however, there is no consensus about performing SG in patients with pre-existing GERD [57].

There are conflicting data about the influence of AGB on GERD [21]. A systematic review [58] reported a decline in the prevalence of postoperative GERD compared to preoperative GERD (7.7 vs. 32.9%) after AGB. The need for anti-reflux medications (9.5 versus 27.5%), pathologic reflux (29.4 versus 55.8%), and lower esophageal pressure (16.9 versus 12.9 mmHg), all decreased in patients who underwent AGB. Fifteen percent of the individuals reported de-novo reflux symptoms.

In short, RYGB is a better option in individuals with uncontrolled severe GERD or Barrett's esophagus.

2.5.3 Joint pain and physical activity

Bariatric surgery could ease joint pain and improve physical activity by reducing weight and inflammation. An observational cohort study reported significant improvement in body pains [57.6% (95% CI, 55.3%–59.9%)], physical function [76.5% (95% CI, 74.6%–78.5%)] & walk time [59.5% (95% CI, 56.4%–62.7%)] at 1 year[59]. However, most of the above symptoms relapsed between 1 and 3 years.

A systematic review showed knee pain improvement in 73% of patients after bariatric surgery [60]. An increase in the intervertebral disc height after successful bariatric surgery was reported in a prospective study [61].

A small prospective study demonstrated a reduction in pro-inflammatory markers (Interleukin 6, C-reactive protein and fibrinogen) after bariatric surgery [62]. This effect could be partly responsible for the improvement in arthritis pain.

2.6 Polycystic ovary syndrome (PCOS)

Obesity is associated with PCOS. Observational studies have reported improved PCOS symptoms (hirsutism, menstrual irregularities and hyperandrogenemia) after bariatric surgery [63, 64].

2.7 Renal disorders

Obesity-related renal impairment could be due to hyperfiltration or other comorbidities such as T2DM, HTN, etc. Another prospective study showed improvement in eGFR 12 months after bariatric surgery [65].

A randomized trial of 100 patients with diabetic nephropathy reported remission of nephropathy in 82 with RYGB vs. 48% with medical therapy at 2 years [66].

Obesity-related urinary incontinence improved after bariatric surgery in the longitudinal assessment of bariatric surgery study [67]. Improvement was maintained at 3 years follow up (24.8%, 95% CI, 21.8%–26.5% among females and 12.2%, 95% CI, 9.0%–16.4% among male).

2.8 Non-alcoholic fatty liver disease (NAFLD)

The prevalence of NAFLD is high in obesity. Non-alcoholic fatty liver disease is treated by lifestyle changes and weight loss [68]. However, bariatric surgery could be considered in cases that failed to improve with medical therapy. A retrospective study of biopsy-proven fibrotic non-alcoholic steatohepatitis reported a lower cumulative incidence of major adverse liver outcomes at 10 years was 2.3% (95% CI, 0%–4.6%) in the surgery group vs. 9.6% (95% CI, 6.1%–12.9%) in the control group [69]. Another database study [70] reported a lower risk of developing cirrhosis in non-alcoholic fatty liver disease patients who underwent bariatric surgery (HR 0.31, 95% CI: 0.19–0.52).

2.9 Mental health issues

Depression (19%) and binge eating disorder (17%) are the most common mental health conditions in the obese population.

Studies have shown improvement in mental health after bariatric surgery. A systematic review [71] reported a decrease in prevalence (8–74%) and severity (40–70%) of depression after bariatric surgery compared to before surgery.

Studies show contradictory reports about the influence of bariatric surgery on eating disorders. A retrospective study reported a durable decline in the loss of control of eating (5.4% post-RYGB vs. 16.2% before surgery), picking/nibbling (7.0% post-RYGB vs. 32.4% before surgery) and craving (19.4% 7 years post-RYGB vs. 33.6% before surgery) [72].

Another study [73] showed a decrease in binge eating disorder in the first two years from 6.1 to 1.3%, but it increased to 3.1% in 3 years.

A large retrospective study [49] reported a higher rate of suicides after RYGB (11.1 vs. 6.4 per 10,000 person-years, P = 0.04). Another large longitudinal cohort study [74] reported a 5-fold increase in deliberate self-harm (incidence rate ratio 4.7; 95% CI, 3.8–5.7). Suicide was reported in 9.6% of cases.

Moreover, studies have shown a high prevalence of alcohol and illicit drug abuse after bariatric surgery. King and Chen [75] observed higher incident alcohol use disorder (AUD) symptoms, substance use and illicit drug abuse after RYGB. Interestingly, the risk of incident AUD was twice higher with RYGB than LAGB.

2.10 Cost-effectiveness

Bariatric surgery is cost-effective in the long run. The cost is higher in the first year than medical treatment and lifestyle changes; however, it is amortized after 3.5 years of surgery [76].

A cost-effective analysis [77] comparing five different weight management programs concluded that in the National Health Service (NHS), RYGB is the most cost-effective surgery.

3. Conclusion

Bariatric surgery is a cost-effective, durable and safe option for managing severe obesity. It confers significant and lasting weight loss. Moreover, the benefit of bariatric surgery extends beyond weight loss. Most obesity-related comorbidities improve after bariatric surgery; remission of T2DM is noteworthy. The indications of bariatric surgery are widening. Some centers advocate bariatric surgery in cases with milder obesity and comorbidities, especially metabolic syndrome. For the long-term success of bariatric surgery, it is essential to couple it with lifestyle changes. Studies have raised concerns about the worsening of mental health problems. It needs close monitoring of high-risk patients and further research.

Acknowledgements

I acknowledge the efforts and support of my master's program tutors from the University of South Wales. They did not contribute to this work directly; however, without their help, completing this work would have been difficult.

I would also like to acknowledge the support from my parents, wife and children while completing this piece of work.

Conflict of interest

The authors declare no conflict of interest.

Notes/thanks/other declarations

None.

Author details

Asad Ullah
King Faisal Specialist Hospital and Research Centre, Riyadh,
Kingdom of Saudi Arabia

*Address all correspondence to: drasadullah99@hotmail.com

References

[1] WHO. Obesity and Overweight 2021 [updated 09-06-2021]. 2021. Available from: https://www.who.int/news-room/fact-sheets/detail/obesity-and-overweight

[2] Nguyen NT, Masoomi H, Magno CP, Nguyen XM, Laugenour K, Lane J. Trends in use of bariatric surgery, 2003-2008. Journal of the American College of Surgeons. 2011;**213**(2):261-266

[3] Arterburn DE, Telem DA, Kushner RF, Courcoulas AP. Benefits and risks of bariatric surgery in adults: A review. Journal of the American Medical Association. 2020;**324**(9):879-887

[4] Brethauer SA, Kim J, el Chaar M, Papasavas P, Eisenberg D, Rogers A, et al. Standardized outcomes reporting in metabolic and bariatric surgery. Surgery for Obesity and Related Diseases. 2015;**11**(3):489-506

[5] Halls S. Metropolitan Life Tables for Women and Men. 2019. Available from: https://halls.md/met-life-ideal-weight/

[6] Devine B. Gentamicin therapy. Drug Intelligence & Clinical Pharmacy. 1974;**8**:650-655

[7] Buchwald H, Avidor Y, Braunwald E, Jensen MD, Pories W, Fahrbach K, et al. Bariatric surgery: A systematic review and meta-analysis. Journal of the American Medical Association. 2004;**292**(14):1724-1737

[8] Peterli R, Borbély Y, Kern B, Gass M, Peters T, Thurnheer M, et al. Early results of the Swiss Multicentre Bypass or Sleeve Study (SM-BOSS): A prospective randomized trial comparing laparoscopic sleeve gastrectomy and Roux-en-Y gastric bypass. Annals of Surgery. 2013;**258**(5):690-694

[9] Grönroos S, Helmiö M, Juuti A, Tiusanen R, Hurme S, Löyttyniemi E, et al. Effect of laparoscopic sleeve gastrectomy vs Roux-en-Y gastric bypass on weight loss and quality of life at 7 years in patients with morbid obesity: The SLEEVEPASS Randomized Clinical Trial. JAMA Surgery. 2021;**156**(2):137-146

[10] Arterburn D, Wellman R, Emiliano A, Smith SR, Odegaard AO, Murali S, et al. Comparative effectiveness and safety of bariatric procedures for weight loss: A PCORnet Cohort Study. Annals of Internal Medicine. 2018;**169**(11):741-750

[11] Ahmed B, King WC, Gourash W, Belle SH, Hinerman A, Pomp A, et al. Long-term weight change and health outcomes for sleeve gastrectomy (SG) and matched Roux-en-Y gastric bypass (RYGB) participants in the Longitudinal Assessment of Bariatric Surgery (LABS) study. Surgery. 2018;**164**(4):774-783

[12] Courcoulas AP, King WC, Belle SH, Berk P, Flum DR, Garcia L, et al. Seven-year weight trajectories and health outcomes in the longitudinal assessment of bariatric surgery (LABS) study. JAMA Surgery. 2018;**153**(5):427-434

[13] Sjöström L. Review of the key results from the Swedish Obese Subjects (SOS) trial - a prospective controlled intervention study of bariatric surgery. Journal of Internal Medicine. 2013;**273**(3):219-234

[14] Maciejewski ML, Arterburn DE, Van Scoyoc L, Smith VA, Yancy WS Jr, Weidenbacher HJ, et al. Bariatric surgery

and long-term durability of weight loss. JAMA Surgery. 2016;**151**(11):1046-1055

[15] Schauer PR, Nor Hanipah Z, Rubino F. Metabolic surgery for treating type 2 diabetes mellitus: Now supported by the world's leading diabetes organizations. Cleveland Clinic Journal of Medicine. 2017;**84**(7 Suppl 1):S47-s56

[16] Rubino F. Is type 2 diabetes an operable intestinal disease? A provocative yet reasonable hypothesis. Diabetes Care. 2008;**31**(Suppl 2):S290-S296

[17] Rhee NA, Vilsbøll T, Knop FK. Current evidence for a role of GLP-1 in Roux-en-Y gastric bypass-induced remission of type 2 diabetes. Diabetes, Obesity & Metabolism. 2012;**14**(4):291-298

[18] Bailly L, Schiavo L, Sebastianelli L, Fabre R, Morisot A, Pradier C, et al. Preventive effect of bariatric surgery on type 2 diabetes onset in morbidly obese inpatients: A national French survey between 2008 and 2016 on 328,509 morbidly obese patients. Surgery for Obesity and Related Diseases. 2019;**15**(3):478-487

[19] Cui BB, Wang GH, Li PZ, Li WZ, Zhu LY, Zhu SH. Long-term outcomes of Roux-en-Y gastric bypass versus medical therapy for patients with type 2 diabetes: A meta-analysis of randomized controlled trials. Surgery for Obesity and Related Diseases. 2021;**17**(7):1334-1343

[20] Buchwald H, Estok R, Fahrbach K, Banel D, Jensen MD, Pories WJ, et al. Weight and type 2 diabetes after bariatric surgery: Systematic review and meta-analysis. The American Journal of Medicine. 2009;**122**(3):248-56.e5

[21] Hutter MM, Schirmer BD, Jones DB, Ko CY, Cohen ME, Merkow RP, et al. First report from the American College of Surgeons Bariatric Surgery Center Network: Laparoscopic sleeve gastrectomy has morbidity and effectiveness positioned between the band and the bypass. Annals of Surgery. 2011;**254**(3):410-420

[22] Salminen P, Helmiö M, Ovaska J, Juuti A, Leivonen M, Peromaa-Haavisto P, et al. Effect of laparoscopic sleeve gastrectomy vs Laparoscopic Roux-en-Y gastric bypass on weight loss at 5 years among patients with morbid obesity: The SLEEVEPASS Randomized Clinical Trial. Journal of the American Medical Association. 2018;**319**(3):241-254

[23] Thereaux J, Lesuffleur T, Czernichow S, Basdevant A, Msika S, Nocca D, et al. Association between bariatric surgery and rates of continuation, discontinuation, or initiation of antidiabetes treatment 6 years later. JAMA Surgery. 2018;**153**(6):526-533

[24] Schauer PR, Kashyap SR, Wolski K, Brethauer SA, Kirwan JP, Pothier CE, et al. Bariatric surgery versus intensive medical therapy in obese patients with diabetes. The New England Journal of Medicine. 2012;**366**(17):1567-1576

[25] Mingrone G, Panunzi S, De Gaetano A, Guidone C, Iaconelli A, Leccesi L, et al. Bariatric surgery versus conventional medical therapy for type 2 diabetes. The New England Journal of Medicine. 2012;**366**(17):1577-1585

[26] Fisher DP, Johnson E, Haneuse S, Arterburn D, Coleman KJ, O'Connor PJ, et al. Association between bariatric surgery and macrovascular disease outcomes in patients with Type 2 diabetes and severe obesity. Journal of the American Medical Association. 2018;**320**(15):1570-1582

[27] Aminian A, Zajichek A, Arterburn DE, Wolski KE, Brethauer SA,

Schauer PR, et al. Association of metabolic surgery with major adverse cardiovascular outcomes in patients with Type 2 diabetes and obesity. Journal of the American Medical Association. 2019;**322**(13):1271-1282

[28] Billeter AT, Eichel S, Scheurlen KM, Probst P, Kopf S, Müller-Stich BP. Meta-analysis of metabolic surgery versus medical treatment for macrovascular complications and mortality in patients with type 2 diabetes. Surgery for Obesity and Related Diseases. 2019;**15**(7):1197-1210

[29] O'Brien R, Johnson E, Haneuse S, Coleman KJ, O'Connor PJ, Fisher DP, et al. Microvascular outcomes in patients with diabetes after bariatric surgery versus usual care: A Matched Cohort Study. Annals of Internal Medicine. 2018;**169**(5):300-310

[30] Holman RR, Paul SK, Bethel MA, Matthews DR, Neil HA. 10-year follow-up of intensive glucose control in type 2 diabetes. The New England Journal of Medicine. 2008;**359**(15):1577-1589

[31] Rubino F, Nathan DM, Eckel RH, Schauer PR, Alberti KG, Zimmet PZ, et al. Metabolic surgery in the treatment algorithm for Type 2 diabetes: A Joint Statement by International Diabetes Organizations. Obesity Surgery. 2017;**27**(1):2-21

[32] Obesity management for the treatment of Type 2 diabetes: Standards of Medical Care in Diabetes-2018. Diabetes Care. 2018;**41**(Suppl 1):S65-s72

[33] Schiavon CA, Bersch-Ferreira AC, Santucci EV, Oliveira JD, Torreglosa CR, Bueno PT, et al. Effects of bariatric surgery in obese patients with hypertension: The GATEWAY randomized trial (gastric bypass to treat obese patients with steady hypertension). Circulation. 2018;**137**(11):1132-1142

[34] Jakobsen GS, Småstuen MC, Sandbu R, Nordstrand N, Hofsø D, Lindberg M, et al. Association of bariatric surgery vs Medical obesity treatment with long-term medical complications and obesity-related comorbidities. Journal of the American Medical Association. 2018;**319**(3):291-301

[35] Zhang N, Maffei A, Cerabona T, Pahuja A, Omana J, Kaul A. Reduction in obesity-related comorbidities: Is gastric bypass better than sleeve gastrectomy? Surgical Endoscopy. 2013;**27**(4):1273-1280

[36] Lee Y, Doumouras AG, Yu J, Aditya I, Gmora S, Anvari M, et al. Laparoscopic Sleeve Gastrectomy Versus Laparoscopic Roux-en-Y Gastric Bypass: A systematic review and meta-analysis of weight loss, comorbidities, and biochemical outcomes from randomized controlled trials. Annals of Surgery. 2021;**273**(1):66-74

[37] Hu Z, Sun J, Li R, Wang Z, Ding H, Zhu T, et al. A comprehensive comparison of LRYGB and LSG in obese patients including the effects on QoL, comorbidities, weight loss, and complications: A systematic review and meta-analysis. Obesity Surgery. 2020;**30**(3):819-827

[38] Ikramuddin S, Korner J, Lee WJ, Connett JE, Inabnet WB, Billington CJ, et al. Roux-en-Y gastric bypass vs intensive medical management for the control of type 2 diabetes, hypertension, and hyperlipidemia: The Diabetes Surgery Study randomized clinical trial. Journal of the American Medical Association. 2013;**309**(21):2240-2249

[39] Nguyen NT, Varela E, Sabio A, Tran CL, Stamos M, Wilson SE. Resolution of hyperlipidemia after laparoscopic Roux-en-Y gastric bypass. Journal of the American College of Surgeons. 2006;**203**(1):24-29

[40] Basen-Engquist K, Chang M. Obesity and cancer risk: Recent review and evidence. Current Oncology Reports. 2011;**13**(1):71-76

[41] Ghiassi S, El Chaar M, Aleassa EM, Moustarah F, El Djouzi S, Birriel TJ, et al. ASMBS position statement on the relationship between obesity and cancer, and the role of bariatric surgery: Risk, timing of treatment, effects on disease biology, and qualification for surgery. Surgery for Obesity and Related Diseases. 2020;**16**(6):713-724

[42] Bardou M, Barkun AN, Martel M. Obesity and colorectal cancer. Gut. 2013;**62**(6):933-947

[43] Mackenzie H, Markar SR, Askari A, Faiz O, Hull M, Purkayastha S, et al. Obesity surgery and risk of cancer. The British Journal of Surgery. 2018;**105**(12):1650-1657

[44] Schauer DP, Feigelson HS, Koebnick C, Caan B, Weinmann S, Leonard AC, et al. Bariatric surgery and the risk of cancer in a large multisite Cohort. Annals of Surgery. 2019;**269**(1):95-101

[45] Bailly L, Fabre R, Pradier C, Iannelli A. Colorectal cancer risk following bariatric surgery in a Nationwide Study of French individuals with obesity. JAMA Surgery. 2020;**155**(5):395-402

[46] Taube M, Peltonen M, Sjöholm K, Anveden Å, Andersson-Assarsson JC, Jacobson P, et al. Association of bariatric surgery with skin cancer incidence in adults with obesity: A Nonrandomized Controlled Trial. JAMA Dermatology. 2020;**156**(1):38-43

[47] Carlsson LMS, Sjöholm K, Jacobson P, Andersson-Assarsson JC, Svensson PA, Taube M, et al. Life expectancy after bariatric surgery in the Swedish Obese Subjects Study. The New England Journal of Medicine. 2020;**383**(16):1535-1543

[48] Doumouras AG, Hong D, Lee Y, Tarride JE, Paterson JM, Anvari M. Association between bariatric surgery and all-cause mortality: A population-based matched Cohort Study in a Universal Health Care System. Annals of Internal Medicine. 2020;**173**(9):694-703

[49] Adams TD, Gress RE, Smith SC, Halverson RC, Simper SC, Rosamond WD, et al. Long-term mortality after gastric bypass surgery. The New England Journal of Medicine. 2007;**357**(8):753-761

[50] Furlan SF, Drager LF, Santos RN, Damiani LP, Bersch-Ferreira AC, Miranda TA, et al. Three-year effects of bariatric surgery on obstructive sleep apnea in patients with obesity grade 1 and 2: A sub-analysis of the GATEWAY trial. International Journal of Obesity. 2021;**45**(4):914-917

[51] Sarkhosh K, Switzer NJ, El-Hadi M, Birch DW, Shi X, Karmali S. The impact of bariatric surgery on obstructive sleep apnea: A systematic review. Obesity Surgery. 2013;**23**(3):414-423

[52] Wong AM, Barnes HN, Joosten SA, Landry SA, Dabscheck E, Mansfield DR, et al. The effect of surgical weight loss on obstructive sleep apnoea: A systematic review and meta-analysis. Sleep Medicine Reviews. 2018;**42**:85-99

[53] Herbella FA, Sweet MP, Tedesco P, Nipomnick I, Patti MG.

Gastroesophageal reflux disease and obesity. Pathophysiology and implications for treatment. Journal of Gastrointestinal Surgery. 2007;**11**(3):286-290

[54] Madalosso CA, Gurski RR, Callegari-Jacques SM, Navarini D, Thiesen V, Fornari F. The impact of gastric bypass on gastroesophageal reflux disease in patients with morbid obesity: A prospective study based on the Montreal Consensus. Annals of Surgery. 2010;**251**(2):244-248

[55] DuPree CE, Blair K, Steele SR, Martin MJ. Laparoscopic sleeve gastrectomy in patients with preexisting gastroesophageal reflux disease : A national analysis. JAMA Surgery. 2014;**149**(4):328-334

[56] Chiu S, Birch DW, Shi X, Sharma AM, Karmali S. Effect of sleeve gastrectomy on gastroesophageal reflux disease: A systematic review. Surgery for Obesity and Related Diseases. 2011;**7**(4):510-515

[57] Rosenthal RJ, Diaz AA, Arvidsson D, Baker RS, Basso N, Bellanger D, et al. International Sleeve Gastrectomy Expert Panel Consensus Statement: Best practice guidelines based on experience of >12,000 cases. Surgery for Obesity and Related Diseases. 2012;**8**(1):8-19

[58] de Jong JR, Besselink MG, van Ramshorst B, Gooszen HG, Smout AJ. Effects of adjustable gastric banding on gastroesophageal reflux and esophageal motility: A systematic review. Obesity Reviews. 2010;**11**(4):297-305

[59] King WC, Chen JY, Belle SH, Courcoulas AP, Dakin GF, Elder KA, et al. Change in pain and physical function following bariatric surgery for severe obesity. Journal of the American Medical Association. 2016;**315**(13):1362-1371

[60] Groen VA, van de Graaf VA, Scholtes VA, Sprague S, van Wagensveld BA, Poolman RW. Effects of bariatric surgery for knee complaints in (morbidly) obese adult patients: A systematic review. Obesity Reviews. 2015;**16**(2):161-170

[61] Lidar Z, Behrbalk E, Regev GJ, Salame K, Keynan O, Schweiger C, et al. Intervertebral disc height changes after weight reduction in morbidly obese patients and its effect on quality of life and radicular and low back pain. Spine (Phila Pa 1976). 2012;**37**(23):1947-1952

[62] Richette P, Poitou C, Garnero P, Vicaut E, Bouillot JL, Lacorte JM, et al. Benefits of massive weight loss on symptoms, systemic inflammation and cartilage turnover in obese patients with knee osteoarthritis. Annals of the Rheumatic Diseases. 2011;**70**(1):139-144

[63] Eid GM, Cottam DR, Velcu LM, Mattar SG, Korytkowski MT, Gosman G, et al. Effective treatment of polycystic ovarian syndrome with Roux-en-Y gastric bypass. Surgery for Obesity and Related Diseases. 2005;**1**(2):77-80

[64] Eid GM, McCloskey C, Titchner R, Korytkowski M, Gross D, Grabowski C, et al. Changes in hormones and biomarkers in polycystic ovarian syndrome treated with gastric bypass. Surgery for Obesity and Related Diseases. 2014;**10**(5):787-791

[65] Hou CC, Shyu RS, Lee WJ, Ser KH, Lee YC, Chen SC. Improved renal function 12 months after bariatric surgery. Surgery for Obesity and Related Diseases. 2013;**9**(2):202-206

[66] Cohen RV, Pereira TV, Aboud CM, Petry TBZ, Lopes Correa JL, Schiavon CA, et al. Effect of gastric bypass vs best medical treatment on early-stage chronic kidney disease

in patients with Type 2 diabetes and obesity: A Randomized Clinical Trial. JAMA Surgery. 2020;**155**(8):e200420

[67] Subak LL, King WC, Belle SH, Chen JY, Courcoulas AP, Ebel FE, et al. Urinary incontinence before and after bariatric surgery. JAMA Internal Medicine. 2015;**175**(8):1378-1387

[68] Day CP. Non-alcoholic fatty liver disease: Current concepts and management strategies. Clinical Medicine (London, England). 2006;**6**(1):19-25

[69] Aminian A, Al Kurd A, Wilson R, Bena J, Fayazzadeh H, Singh T, et al. Association of bariatric surgery with major adverse liver and cardiovascular outcomes in patients with biopsy-proven nonalcoholic steatohepatitis. Journal of the American Medical Association. 2021;**326**(20):2031-2042

[70] Hafeez S, Ahmed MH. Bariatric surgery as potential treatment for nonalcoholic fatty liver disease: A future treatment by choice or by chance? Journal of Obesity. 2013;**2013**:839275

[71] Dawes AJ, Maggard-Gibbons M, Maher AR, Booth MJ, Miake-Lye I, Beroes JM, et al. Mental health conditions among patients seeking and undergoing bariatric surgery: A meta-analysis. Journal of the American Medical Association. 2016;**315**(2):150-163

[72] Devlin MJ, King WC, Kalarchian MA, Hinerman A, Marcus MD, Yanovski SZ, et al. Eating pathology and associations with long-term changes in weight and quality of life in the longitudinal assessment of bariatric surgery study. The International Journal of Eating Disorders. 2018;**51**(12):1322-1330

[73] Kalarchian MA, King WC, Devlin MJ, Marcus MD, Garcia L, Chen JY, et al. Psychiatric disorders and weight change in a prospective study of bariatric surgery patients: A 3-year follow-up. Psychosomatic Medicine. 2016;**78**(3):373-381

[74] Morgan DJR, Ho KM, Platell C. Incidence and determinants of mental health service use after bariatric surgery. JAMA Psychiatry. 2020;**77**(1):60-67

[75] King WC, Chen JY, Courcoulas AP, Dakin GF, Engel SG, Flum DR, et al. Alcohol and other substance use after bariatric surgery: Prospective evidence from a U.S. multicenter cohort study. Surgery for Obesity and Related Diseases. 2017;**13**(8):1392-1402

[76] Sampalis JS, Liberman M, Auger S, Christou NV. The impact of weight reduction surgery on health-care costs in morbidly obese patients. Obesity Surgery. 2004;**14**(7):939-947

[77] Boyers D, Retat L, Jacobsen E, Avenell A, Aveyard P, Corbould E, et al. Cost-effectiveness of bariatric surgery and non-surgical weight management programmes for adults with severe obesity: A decision analysis model. International Journal of Obesity. 2021;**45**(10):2179-2190